THE AGE OF WAITING

ARROWSMITH
PRESS

The Age of Waiting
Douglas J. Penick
© 2020 Arrowsmith Press
All Rights Reserved

ISBN: 978-1-7346416-4-6

Boston — New York — San Francisco — Baghdad
San Juan — Kyiv — Istanbul — Santiago, Chile
Beijing — Paris — London — Cairo — Madrid
Milan — Melbourne — Jerusalem — Darfur

11 Chestnut St.
Medford, MA 02155

arrowsmithpress@gmail.com
www.arrowsmithpress.com

The thirty-third Arrowsmith book was typeset & designed
by Ezra Fox for Askold Melnyczuk & Alex Johnson
in Trajan Pro & Optima typefaces

Cover image: Albrecht Dürer's Traumgesicht (Dream Vision)
(Note: this image is referenced on page 104)

Essays in this book first appeared in various foms in the following publications:

A World Ever at its End — *Tricycle*, summer 2017 | A Vanished Buddhist King —
Tricycle, spring 2018 | A Telephone Call —— *Shambhala Sun*, May 2014 | Encountering
Old Age —— *Tricycle*, fall 2015 | Sickness —— *Tricycle*, winter 2015 | Death —— *Tricycle*,
spring 2016 | Path —— *Tricycle*, summer 2016 | The Empty Room (originally By The
River) —— *Annak Sastra*, issue 7 | Die Gleise (The Tracks) —— *Consequence Magazine*,
fall 2019 | Paths in Gathering Darkness (originally Exploring What Is) —— *Tricycle*,
fall 2018 | A Vanished Sage —— *Tricycle*, summer 2018 | For Music —— *Tricycle*,
winter 2020 | Noble Heart of All Existence —— *Shambhala Sun*, September 2008

THE AGE OF WAITING

HEART TRACES
&
SONG LINES IN THE ANTHROPOCENE

Douglas J. Penick

CONTENTS

FOREWORD

"We have been living in a blind alley...dominated by the feeling 'it cannot last.'"

— Victor Serge

The jungles of legend with their brilliantly colored birds, green shimmering rivers, glittering serpents, iridescent butterflies, black leopards waiting like animate shadows; the radiant undersea reefs, multicolored, alive with darting fish of strange shapes and coloration; the remote bluish silence of the vast arctic ice; as a child, I saw such images in magazines and movies. Those who brought us evidence of such distant and magical worlds were heroes. One day, I almost dared to hope, I might actually experience visions of such intensity. Now, in the same magazines, in new images online and on TV, it is different. The world's vividness is fading before our eyes. We see polluted seas, ruined forests, empty deserts. We read how corporations exploit the wonders of the world. We read a litany of extinctions. We see the glaciers shrink. We are offered a bleak future with mass starvation, mass migration, and new plagues. We are hearing about the end of a long story. And we can only wait.

The landscape of our world now is overwhelmed by human activity and human construction. We have developed technologies for making use of an unimaginable range of natural resources, and for enhancing, diminishing, and diverting human desires. These technologies have allowed for immense increases in human population at the expense of the integrity of the natural world. Many now call our time the Anthropocene: the time when humanity's influence is deciding the shape and fate of the earth and its occupants. Human domination has now led to ever greater destruction and pollution of the natural world.

We find ourselves powerless to reverse the course of our own destruction. Our habits of mind have too narrow a focus. We cannot join together in the kinds of global cooperation needed to prevent catastrophe. We cannot make the individual sacrifices needed for such an effort. We cannot subordinate our national interests to a global need. Our politicians turn away from science and join with leaders of the corporate economy to deny the scientific conclusions which have previously supported their practices, and seek only to increase the level of world exploitation. No one knows how to think in any other way. Our era, the Anthropocene, the era of a world man-made, is not a time of optimism. It seems our journey on the earth has been oblivious. Burdened by apprehension, we wait. As we wait, we move this way and that, revisiting old possibilities, listening for messages from other times.

"It was the human longing to connect, to see patterns no matter how the dots are scattered."

— Robert Karjel

Long ago, before history, the ancestors of the original people in Australia sang the world, its mountains, rivers, deserts, trees, its mammals, birds, and lizards, into existence. This took place in what humans called the dream time.

In dreams, people and tribes recognized their identity with the land, their animal, bird, lizard, and insect predecessors, and recognized a specific inner relationship with those animals, birds, lizards, and insects today. From their fellow men and women, from what they heard in dreams, they learned the songs of the landscape, the sky, the dreamtime, the deeds of their human and non-human predecessors. When people and tribes moved across the landscape, they sang these songs. Singing and travelling were synchronized, and enabled them to survive. A vast and evolving pattern was weaving itself. Moving along the song lines which crisscross the continent, women and men continually unified spirit and human worlds, past and present time, and in this unbroken continuity they have known their way.

Now, in the rest of the world, the many song lines that map the globe are almost inaudible. When we try to listen for intuitions of a spiritual path, guidance from the past, stories of our forebears, we find it is like walking through a huge apartment building in a big city. The din of automobiles, subways, airplanes, televised mass-media, recorded music, men and women shouting, children crying, cell phones beeping, is deafening. Yet, subtler promptings are not entirely drowned out.

Hints, clues, images, fragments of thought, fragments of dreams, remembered smells, half-forgotten music, and minute promptings point the way towards a possibility we cannot quite articulate. Teachings, poems, music, and stories open doors we still cannot quite enter. Lost, deep within the world that humans have made and are making, we still sense promptings that might lead to other ways of seeing, ways of proceeding that are now only vaguely imagined, patterns that are not quite accessible. We wander through the world, waiting to hear the whispers that will open in our heart.

"Just take a little leap after that. ... That's it!"

– Chögyam Trungpa Rinpoche

A WORLD EVER AT ITS END

I

I look out the window at the foothills of the Rocky Mountains. Recent floods have scarred their flanks. Deep pine forests that once cascaded luxuriantly over the crests are thinning out. Now, patches of pine trees, attacked by the mountain pine beetle, die and turn a strangely violent rust color. As if burned, they become black and ashy. The forest's silhouette, running from peak to peak, is no longer soft and verdant. Spikes of skeletal trunks and branches scratch at the sky. It's a sign: the world we know is moving to its end.

The warmer weather, scientists say, *the diminished periods of deep cold.* More larvae of pine beetles now survive. And now, if we drive deeper into the mountains, we pass through vast swaths of dead forest — brittle, gray, black — almost indistinguishable from the acres and acres decimated by summer forest fires that recently lit up the night skies. I cannot bear to drive there now.

These are echoes of what we see on television and read in the papers: melting polar caps, sea glaciers breaking apart, mountain glaciers shrinking; the expanding deserts, the ferocious territorial wars, people covered in hazmat suits helping those stricken with new diseases, streams of desperate migrants by the millions. Scientists predict worse. The civilization we inhabit is beginning to break. We have all heard this. Assumptions and certainties are caving in.

The feeling of being slowly swallowed, anaesthetized. We cannot think how to resist. We watch, horrified, spellbound.

Cold prickles my scalp.
It's forbidden to speak out.
Time cuts me off
As your heel grinds me down.

Life turns against life.
Sound slowly breaks up.
Things drop out of sight
Past remembering in no time.

Oh yes, it once was better.
Please, you can't compare:
Oh my blood, what stirred you then;
O blood, what stirs you now.

Plainly there's some design
Now playing on these lips:
Winds are playing in the treetops
Doomed to be chopped down.

As the jaws of terror that would consume millions began to open in Russia in 1923, Osip Mandelstam wrote this.

II

There is a vast invisible blade of glass; it cuts through the world, and beyond the world. On the surface of this thin transparent plane, we see all that is conceivable, imaginable, perceptible. We are looking at a vast shimmering mural. Its beginning and end are unknowable.

We may think of this transparent plane as consciousness, or as awareness, or as any other way of knowing.

What appears on this plane is a reduction of vaster and more unknowable realities for which our mind provides no set of references. These are sights beyond the spectra we can see, music beyond sounds anyone can hear, and patterns anyone can comprehend; they are harmonies beyond form, language beyond grammar and words, knowing beyond consciousness, intensities beyond the framework of heart, brain, senses, and nerves.

The Buddha pointed at this and beyond.

A consort of Emperor Sushun sang:

Higher than the king's house,
Finer than silk.
Indivisible.
Ungraspable as smoke.

III

Stories from innumerable human cultures tell of a moment when the presiding deity wearied of the greedy, self-centered dealings of men and women, of the corruption they have inflicted on society and the world. The deity, whoever she or he might be, then sent a great flood to purify the earth. Rains descended, rivers and lakes overflowed, oceans and seas covered the land. Humanity with all its spoiled and ungrateful megalomania was washed away.

And though humanity has repeatedly returned, whether from flood or drought, from fire or war or plague, it has always again fallen. Now the landscape of our passage on the earth is a diorama of ruins of great cities, strange funerary monuments, half-forgotten philosophies, outlines of gardens, broken amphitheaters, nameless corpses, ruined palaces, fragmentary poetry, lyrics without music, spiritual paths without practitioners, libraries without books. Our time on earth is recorded in what remains of histories and innumerable epics where kings, heroes, and warrior queens lead their people into battle, fight to conquer or resist conquest, enslave or become enslaved, destroy worlds and see worlds destroyed.

In Hindu and Buddhist traditions it is maintained that existence moves continuously through cycles of increase and decrease, expansion and contraction, waxing and waning. These cycles are divided into eras called the four Yugas. The first, the Satya Yuga, is the longest and most ideal, a time of inner and outer beauty, purity, and perfection. Desires and their fulfillment arise simultaneously. It is said to last 1,728,000 years. Next is the Treta Yuga of 1,296,000 years. In this era, perfection begins to wane slightly. Longings, paths, and goals begin to unravel. In the Dvapara Yuga that lasts 864,000 years, desires, intentions, actions, and social classes become ever more distinct and varied. Finally, there is our era, the shortest, the Kali Yuga, a time of destruction lasting 432,000 years.

Now, in the Kali Yuga, desire and the objects of desire have separated. We struggle to join them, but the results are temporary. Even our cravings themselves are momentary, marked by anguish, longing, and rage. Spiritual, moral, and ethical life degenerates. Material advantage becomes our only value. Pollution, corruption, disease, degeneration, and violence fill our minds, poisoning the world. The only virtue that can still be practiced is compassion. We are moving into the end of time. All will end before another cycle begins.

And indeed, we feel the end approaching. The tempo of mass destruction has increased. The last century saw unparalleled slaughter, destruction, and dislocation; it saw two world wars, internal slaughters in China, Russia, Cambodia, Uganda, the atom bomb, the Holocaust, and innumerable other episodes of mass violence. Dread and unreality now pervade the mind-stream of the age.

IV

Jorge Semprún, a Spanish resistance agent in Paris, was arrested by the Gestapo in 1943. He spent the remainder of the war in the kingdom of the dead known as Buchenwald. Upon his release, he found the world of normal living an alien terrain.

"Death loomed up once again in my future, cunning and inevitable. .... I would then have the precise and crushing impression of living only in a dream. Of being a dream myself. Before dying in Buchenwald, before drifting away in smoke across the Ettersberg, I'd dreamed of this future, this deceptive incarnation."

In the 1970s, Li Zhiwu recounted a fever dream he had as a youth of nineteen while lying in bed during the famine precipitated by the Great Leap Forward. His limbs were heavy with edema:

> "I saw two villages, one on this side of a ravine, one on that side. The one on this side looked like my home village. There was a bridge from this side to that side, a single log, narrow and slippery. I was ordered to walk to that side, but I was afraid, and halfway across I fell off. I woke up alive. If I had made it to the other side I would have died… for that other side was the land of death."

The little garden, once hidden and remote in the middle of the city and between tall buildings, was coated with gray dust. My friend could not stop talking. Here, he said, lay thirty-seven bodies that had burned to death in the cellar. "And look, there's a bloody boot." It was a bombproof cellar, but the doors had jammed. And because the coal bin next to it had caught fire, they had all been roasted alive. They had all pushed away from the hot walls to the middle of the cellar. There they were found pressed together, bloated from the heat. "And come up here!" He helped me to climb a hill of rubble there. From the desert that lay before us, only the portal of the Konventgarten was standing. We had heard the Brandenburg Concertos there in April. And a blind woman had sung: "Die schwere Leidenszeit beginnt nun abermals." (The time of suffering now begins once more.)

> "Simple and self-assured, the singer had stood leaning against the harpsichord, and her dead eyes had gazed past the vain things for which we were even then already longing. Perhaps they were gazing at where we stood now."

V

There never was a Golden Age in this, the Kali Yuga. There has never been a life of enduring attainments and lasting peace. Our time, our sense of time, is defined by a struggle to exist, by impermanence, repeated loss, by constant termination. From the beginning, our world has been ending. End over end. Individuals and populations have always experienced the destruction of the world. This is the meaning of Kali Yuga.

Hélène Cixous does not hold back when she says: "... Death gives us the essential primitive experience, access to the other world, which is not without warning or noise...it gives us everything, it gives us the end of the world; to be human, we need to experience the end of the world."

Now indeed we may be in the most global and final version of our repeated extinctions. The earth may no longer endure the burden of overpopulation, the industrial production that provides an ever-larger population with ever-higher standards of material life. Now, perhaps more clearly than ever before, we are looking at the end of time measured in terms of a human generation or life-span of human memory altogether.

But Mme. Cixous continues: "We need to lose the world, to lose a world, and to discover there is more than one world, and that the world isn't what we think it is."

VI

Cheng Man Ch'ing, renowned for his mastery of Tai Chi, calligraphy, medicine, philosophy, and poetry, lived through the unimaginable and final destruction of an imperial system that had lasted five thousand years. He witnessed the birth of the Republic of China, which ended as

China was devoured by warlords and invaders. He escaped the mainland when the Communist Party undertook the complete re-creation of culture. He lived the latter part of his life in exile, and taught what he could.

Once, when teaching martial arts, he paused and said: "If you are standing at the edge of a great precipice, and someone is trying to push you off this cliff, and, if you think you have an enemy, you have made your last mistake."

The Zen teacher Shunryu Suzuki Roshi endured the destruction and rebirth of his homeland. He once instructed his meditation students in this way:

Don't move. Just die. Over and over.
Don't anticipate. Nothing can save you now, because you have only this moment.
Not even enlightenment will help you now, because there are no other moments.
With no future, be true to yourself and express yourself fully.
Don't move.
Just die.
Over and over.

A Western spiritual teacher contracted a fatal disease. He knew he would not escape the destruction of his reputation. "Love never dies," he said. As he was wheeled into the hospital to die, he looked up at one of his few remaining supporters, smiled, winked. "Is this the sad part now?"

VI

It was an unusually warm day in late fall. I was having coffee with an elderly friend. She had expected to die a year ago, had almost died a few other times, and was still subject to recurrences of a rare, lethal, and incurable cancer. Though she was now reliant on the oxygen tank she carried with her, her directness, humor, and momentum were uncompromised. I wanted to ask her about something that she, more than anyone I knew, could address.

For some time, she and I had shared a curious space. My melanoma has been quiescent, but still of the most lethal kind. I had, from the beginning, accepted the worst. So I wanted to know what she made of having accepted the immediate likelihood of being dead while finding oneself continuously and actively alive. I thought the question might interest her.

"Your situation is a lot more immediate than mine, to say the least. But here we are. Living. What do you make of it?"

"It's… it's so odd, really, isn't it? I'm here. I do things I've always enjoyed. I go to concerts. I like this coffee…. The yellow leaves… and yet… it's somehow… maybe… not part of things… I don't know. There's nothing to think, is there?"

A memory suddenly came to mind about my teacher, Trungpa Rinpoche, a Tibetan abbot who had lived more than half his life in exile. I was sitting in the back row. It was shortly before Rinpoche died, and he spoke slowly and deliberately. He ended the talk, saying that the teachings could "resolve the basic duality of human existence."

"And what is the basic duality of human existence?" an alert young woman asked. Trungpa Rinpoche answered with careful emphasis: "The basic duality of human existence is… Cheerful… and….Strange."

The woman hesitated: "What do you mean, Strange?"

Rinpoche smiled warmly. "Oh, you know… étrange."

My friend looked at me, paused a long time, and said: "...I don't know why, but that's actually quite helpful."

She took my hand, gave a little laugh, squeezed, shrugged, looked away.

VII

Do you think this moment is forever gone?
Or was it just an echo of a different time and place?

Briefly,
Do you remember/dream: walking down a corridor.
When was that? Where?

Briefly,
Do you see an old man, silver-haired, dancing across
    the stage;
Elegant, ardent, determined.

Briefly,
A woman cries, her face crumples.

Briefly,
On a cold winter day,
The smell of early spring,
Pink-tinged silver clouds,
The dawn and love.
Briefly,
Do you know
If a painter will pick up a brush.

VIII

Paralyzing August heat. The whole city is sweating. Pedestrians avoid the sides of the street with direct sunlight. I'm in the shadow of an awning drinking ice tea. Across the street, in the glaring heat, an old white man in rags, drunk, rummages in a trash bin, looks up, stares at me furious, insane.

"Hey man." Even from the other side of the street, it's as if he's seeing something in me I don't want to know about. "Yes you, fucker. Now what are you gonna do, huh? It's over. Finished. What you gonna do?"

I want to look at something else, but can't. The old man gives me a demented, toothless leer. He reaches down into the trash, and his hand comes out filled with some lumpy, white, semi-liquid that might be yoghurt. It drips between his blackened fingers as he stuffs it in his mouth, watching me all the while. The white goo runs out of the corners of his mouth. His grin turns again to fury. "Don't look away."

──FOR A TIME A DREAM WOULD TAKE ME

S ometimes people tell us dreams which then become lodged in our imagining. After a while, we come to think the dream was almost our own, and it becomes a fugitive reference point for a moment of awareness we may re-visit. Such a dream was told to me by my friend Edward, a renowned painter, a great raconteur, and a man who prided himself on extreme lucidity. It was late, and we were walking to the subway after a night of drinking. He had been talking for a few hours non-stop about the impending ecological collapse. "People are selfish, frightened. They can't change their basic logic, even if they want to change where it's taking them. It's over. All we can do is wait." This had been his curtain line as we left the bar.

He didn't say anything as we walked along the empty streets. Then he told me a dream he'd often had. It often returned, he said; then it changed, returning in an altered and disappointing form, until finally it vanished.

He'd found himself standing before a narrow brick building in the 1920's Federal style. On a whim, he walked up the three worn granite steps, entered into a shallow alcove, and turned the worn brass handle on an old green wooden door.

Then he was walking down a narrow hallway with brass wall sconces. Then another door, wood painted black. This opened suddenly onto a room with pale gray walls and white trim, cool and evenly bright. Then he was in an old-fashioned academic museum with bronze and glass cases in orderly ranks. There were no visitors, though he heard the hum of voices in an office somewhere. The wood floor creaked as he moved slowly through the frozen panoply of antiquities on display. Mostly these were Greek and Roman, small terra-cotta statues, fragments of faces, pottery, and glass. He drifted along the outer walls, there coming to a brown unmarked metal fire-door. Unmarked. It opened easily, and he entered. Before him an iron staircase rose in a shadowy stairwell. Trying to step softly to muffle the clanking, he climbed up several stories.

Through another door, he entered a large attic. It smelled of dust. He was sure this wasn't open to the public. The room was completely silent, and mostly in shadow. But slowly, as his eyes adjusted, he saw rows of cabinets filled with gilded bronze statues of unfamiliar deities, small solid gold animals, beautiful geometric polychrome vases, stone sculptures of sages, courtesans and rulers. They were all very old, but unlike anything he had seen. The proportions of the figures were elongated, as if gravity had less effect on them. Many of the faces shared an elusive, even secretive expression. There were no labels.

Propped against the wall, in wooden crates, were fragments of faded murals depicting battles, ceremonies, and landscapes. The pigments, only slightly faded, were strange. The purples were more intense, the greens and reds more vivid, the blues deeper than any of the murals he knew. They conveyed an atmosphere of profound and unfamiliar harmony. They were like the remnants of dream worlds. He examined pictures and objects until they all were once again engulfed by sleep.

This dream returned maybe ten times over half as many years. And on each visit to the attic, Edward saw some vase or image not noticed before. But he never could remember exactly. It was an alternative past he couldn't hold on to.

Then, one night, the dream began again as ever, but now the door to the attic store house was gone. The wall was smooth and hard. He couldn't reach the attic now. He returned in dreams a few more times, looking for the door, but it didn't exist. It was a painful disappointment. Eventually the dream ceased.

The memory of Edward's dream drifted back one afternoon when I ventured into a bookstore hidden away on the second floor of a building in midtown. It consisted of two or three huge rooms clogged with iron industrial shelving. The store sold only works from Asia in translation. At the time, it was all completely unfamiliar. But something was reaching out. At random I opened a book. It was a Han dynasty commentary on the *Book of Odes*. The page I had turned to told of an evil Prince who was one day looking west from his palace roof. He turned to his Prime Minister, and declared his intention to invade and destroy his neighbors there. The Prime Minister objected, and the Prince immediately had him beheaded. The commentary on this story insisted that the Prime Minister had been foolish. He should have known that the Prince was an evil man, and he should have preserved his wisdom and talents for a more worthy employer. All this, in turn, was a commentary on a line of poetry that said something like: "Plum blossoms fall amid unseasonable winds."

This train of thought seemed utterly alien. I bought the book, but I was never again able to find this story.

§ § §

*F*rom the time I was four onward, my mother told me stories from all over the world. I would lie on my bed in the shadows. Over her shoulder, the light on the bureau fell on the book she read. I would drift into the worlds that unfolded from her words, and dissolve into those distant realities. My favorite was Scheherazade.

Scheherazade, as everyone one knows, married a king named Shahriyar, a man with such a violent desire and hatred for women that he married a new wife every day and had her killed the next morning. To put an end to this mindless slaughter, Scheherazade roused all her courage and gave herself to King Shahriyar. She had a plan. After their wedding night, Scheherazade asked the King if she might tell him a story. The King, ever restless, agreed.

So began one thousand and one nights and one thousand and one stories. On some nights, Scheherazade told several tales, on others she told stories that took days. But every day, as the sun rose, whatever tale she was telling was not complete, and King Shahriyar postponed her execution. Every day, Scheherazade lived because her husband wanted to hear the rest of the story.

For more than three years, Scheherazade never knew if she would live to see the next day. Every evening she knew she might be killed in a few hours' time. For more than three years she continued to exert the power of her art to preserve her life and the lives of others her husband would, if she failed, marry afterwards.

The innumerable stories that Scheherazade told her homicidal lover (known later as The 1001 Nights) came from Persia, Syria, Byzantium, Arabia, India, Egypt, Morocco, Waziristan, Tunisia, Spain, and many lands between and beyond. They reflected the travels of thousands and thousands of merchants who ventured across vast deserts, through deep mountain ranges, and on uncharted seas. They had risked their lives for adventure and to find their fortunes. Everywhere they traded goods, and in every city and bazaar they traded stories.

In these stories could be found every kind of god and demon, every kind of woman and man, and many kinds of beasts and sea creatures; they were bound together by nets of war, romance, hatred, greed, spiritual seeking, perversion, and love.

But it was not Scheherazade's aim merely to distract the King from his rage, nor to keep him occupied until his passion for her became stronger than his desire to kill her. In Scheherazade's telling, these stories reflected elements of each other, and echoed each other. She wove them together, joining images and themes in a great magic carpet that transported her husband to many unfamiliar places, and showed him many secret worlds.

And did she know she would succeed in changing her fate? No. There was no certainty here. Each night she faced her death. Each night she drew on all her resources of courage and invention. Even so, there was not an instant when the King could not suddenly decide he'd had enough. She would die, and the slaughter would begin again. All she could do was continue.

At first, the King may have postponed his wife's execution out of mere curiosity to find out what happened next. But slowly his imagination came to life as he found himself living lives other than his own, exploring realms he had never before imagined. He encountered unknown peoples who wore strange clothes, spoke unknown languages, had unfamiliar creeds and customs. He entered unfamiliar cities, saw palaces of great beauty, was threatened with dungeons and tortures, diseases and many kinds of death. He faced bandits and corrupt officials, wise men, despots, generous patrons, and women, beauties, shrews, magicians, as well as sea monsters, djinns, genies, animals that could talk, and statues that could kill. Sometimes he was an old man, a child, a bird, a donkey, a woman. Scheherazade's stories changed King Shahriyar. They made him fall in love, and they brought him into a larger world.

For three years, in the strange intimacy of artist and executioner, Scheherazade and King Shahriyar shared hundreds of adventures in hundreds of lands. The story by which we know them became, for them, only one of innumerable possibilities. In that time she bore him three sons. After one thousand and one nights of such journeys, King Shahriyar had been changed. He lifted the sentence of death and prayed aloud: "May God prolong your life and increase your dignity and the awe that you inspire throughout all time."

This is the gift of Scheherazade: a world that is perpetually renewed, that resists and constantly defeats death. In the world of passion and relentless craving, the world of form with its suffering, slaughter, vanity, selfishness, waste, and inescapable death, there is always something within passion itself that opens doors to a different world, and a different way of embracing the world in which we find ourselves. Knowing the story of Scheherazade's stories, knowing that also death stalks us, we do not stop looking, listening, touching, feeling, knowing, searching.

—A VANISHED BUDDHIST KING:

LUBSAN SAMDAN TSYDENOV

Life, the great destroyer, is the source of all.
Compassion, rejecting nothing, has never known fear;
Here is Yamantaka, the Conqueror of Death,
Dwelling inseparably in the center of the gold cloud-palace of the senses:
This is the supreme protection.

§ § §

Like coming upon a worn sandstone sculpture in the remote steppes, the life story of Lubsan Samdan Tsydenov is strangely imposing, even monumental. Its sources are difficult to access, and not entirely easy to verify. He emerges from a confused and violent past, and he seems more a heroic figure in a folktale, like an emanation of Gesar, say, than an actual historical person. But it is undisputed that he was destined to be a monk, that he lived as a Buddhist teacher, that he became a king, and that, finally, he disappeared into the violent chaos of the early 20th century.

It is agreed that Samdan Tsydenov was born in 1850 in southern Buryatia near Lake Baikal. Buryatia is a south-central Siberian territory bordered by Russia to the north, Mongolia to the south, and Lake Baikal to the east. It is the homeland of several Buryat Mongol tribes, and has, since the 18th century, been the northernmost territory to adopt Tibetan Buddhist practices.

Even as a small boy, Tsydenov had a reputation for stubbornness. People still tell the story about his determination. One spring morning he joined a group of children competing to see how far they could throw stones into a broad stream. He was not the best, but long after the others had gone home, Tsydenov remained, pitching one stone after another as far as he could. He continued through the rest of the day and well into the evening. By the time his mother came to find him, the stream was dammed and a small lake had begun to form. The lake remains today, and even if the man himself has been forgotten, it is still called Samdan Lake.

When he was ten, his parents sent him to Kudun Datsan, the nearby Gelugpa Monastery, where it is said his concentration in study and in meditation practice was more single-minded than anyone had ever seen. Once the abbot sent him to bring a mare back from a distant pasture. He was preoccupied in reflecting on the nature of suffering and returned hours later, empty-handed. A farmer had seen Tsydenov walk right past the animal, but when the abbot asked Tsydenov what had happened, Tsydenov replied: "I went to the pasture, as you told me, but there is no horse." Some thought that this reply was evidence of his strict discipline, while others found in it an echo of Bodhidharma's proclamation of shunyata, or emptiness.

Throughout the following years, Tsydenov's meditation practice was unwavering, and he remained an omnivorous scholar. Many accounts assert that he studied Western philosophy when he could find texts, and he sought out traveling Nyingma lamas, followers of the earliest Buddhist teaching in Tibet, for instruction. In this period, Tsydenov also became a disciple of the 13th Jayagsy Gegen Tulku, abbot of the great Kumbum

Monastery in Tibet. Tsydenov was thirty-five when, after years of study, he passed the rigorous tests for the title of Geshe, the equivalent of a philosophy doctorate. At that point, he became an official part of the Buddhist hierarchy in Buryatia.

Jayagsy Tulku made several visits to Buryatia and gave Tsydenov special oral instructions on the practice of Yamantaka, conqueror of the Lord of Death. The two also discussed at great length the future of Buddhist institutions. According to notebooks of people who had spoken with him, Tsydenov believed that the 20th century would bring unparalleled upheavals, and that the monastic way of life would no longer be able to ensure the continuity of the Buddha's teachings. He proposed instead to establish a community of lay practitioners who would focus on older forms of tantric practice. This was the only way, as he later wrote, that the Buddhadharma could survive and even expand to the West. Despite what many have characterized as Tsydenov's aloof manner, his clarity of mind and absolute devotion earned the admiration and trust of the Buddhist community.

It is true, however, that they sometimes found their new Geshe alarming. Once, a wealthy layman requested Tsydenov to perform an offering to Dorje Legpa, a powerful protector (particularly of manufacturers and merchants) frequently shown riding on a goat, wearing a gold helmet, and holding a hammer and bellows. The layman had unfurled a thangka [scroll painting] of the deity above the shrine, and set out rows of ritual offering cakes before it. When Tsydenov arrived, he took down the thangka and rolled it up, then shredded the offerings and scattered them, saying, "Surely, this is more than enough for an ordinary blacksmith." From this, people saw that for Tsydenov, the world of deities and the world of human beings were not separate.

When the abbot of Kunun died, many wanted Tsydenov to be appointed to the position. A clique who resented Tsydenov's gifts and reputation prevented this. He was, however, invited to be one of a party of Buryat nobles and priests invited to visit Moscow to attend the coronation of Nicholas II in May 1896. From scattered accounts, it is possible to infer what followed:

The Buryat delegation attended the coronation of the Assumption Cathedral in Moscow. A later audience took place near St. Petersburg in the long, gilded hall of the imperial palace at Tsarskoye Selo. The guests felt engulfed in the glow of gold plasterwork. Nothing in the way they lived prepared them for the brilliance of the churches and palaces. They were dazzled amid mirrors blazing as if lit from within. It was like being in the center of a sun. The visitors from the remote Siberian steppes had never imagined such splendor on such a scale.

A court functionary in black banged his ivory staff. Guards in silver breastplates snapped to attention, and Nicholas, in a uniform of deep red with gold braid, entered quickly and sat on his silver throne. Everyone was overcome with awe. All bowed low, as instructed, except Tsydenov. He stood, stared at the Tsar, and nodded respectfully. Courtiers and visitors were equally aghast. Tsydenov later maintained that his vows and the Vinaya, the monastic code of rules, did not permit a monk to bow to a secular ruler. The head of the delegation made anxious excuses to court functionaries, saying that Tsydenov had been stunned by the sight of the Tsar and did not know what he was doing. The apology was accepted.

While he was in St. Petersburg and Moscow, Tsydenov met with Western intellectuals and orientalists, from whom he obtained books on Western philosophy and political theory. But when he returned from St. Petersburg, he did not stay long at Kumbum Monastery. "A monastery is also samsara," he said. Accompanied by a few students, he withdrew to the remote village of Soorkhoi and remained there on retreat for more than 20 years.

After the coronation in the early summer of 1896, most surprisingly, Tsydenov sent a poem, written in Tibetan, to the Tsar. It was a long dream-vision of a transcendent ruler in a celestial realm of unimaginable opulence and beauty. Here Nicholas II was seen both as an enlightened monarch, or cakravartin, and an emanation of the deity, White Tara, who spreads peace and wisdom just as a Buddha's wisdom permeates his world. The

Tsarina was presented in the poem as a divine consort, with attendants who lived to fulfill the Tsar's mission in the world.

And so, even if there was a time when Tsydenov would not bow to the Tsar, now we find him writing of Russian cities as if they were filled with the magical beauties of a pure land, and of Nicholas II and his court as worldly deities. Perhaps he sensed how much the world would change, and how the imperial order embodied virtues that would be swept away.

Here is a part of this ode:

Like the full moon amid stars,
The Tsar Nicholas, the radiant Lord, blesses the minds of
    all his subjects.
As he emerges in the sky with his radiant consort,
He embodies the fulfillment of all the world's longings.
. . .
I look up and the sky opens,
And just as the still expanse of the sea
Is suddenly ornamented with shining ripples,
It seems my body is wrapped in golden cloth.
The hair on my skin rises and shivers.
For a long time, I cannot move.
Then I make three prostrations.
I offer the symbols for an enduring life:
A white silk scarf, a jeweled mandala, a statue of Amataeus,
Embodiment of Life and Light.
I pray:
May this ruler forever entrance our minds,
Forever dispel the darkness of disorder and chaos.
May he sit in splendor on his diamond throne.
. . .

May the pure land of imperial rule
Pervade all time.
Without a holy ruler,
How can humankind know peace?
Please protect us from the madness of the world

. . .

May this song, written down under the light of two electric bulbs, bring all-pervasive purity and perfect bliss to every sentient being.

Tsydenov and his followers remained in determined seclusion, but from the beginning of the new century, the world was careening into chaos. All across Russia, in the first decade of the 20th century, people rose up against the crown. At the beginning of the second decade, thousands of years of imperial rule ended in China. In the midst of encroaching chaos, Tsydenov began to study the most ancient tantras, and though still on retreat, was asked to serve as abbot of Kudun Datsan. He accepted the responsibility, but stayed in Soorkhoi while his students looked after the day-to-day management of the monastery. Some years later, when the Buddhist hierarchy demanded it, he was more than happy to surrender both title and work. Everyone had heard that the provisional government in St. Petersburg was failing, and that hundreds of thousands of Russians were being killed on the battlefields of Europe. While the Red Armies campaigned in western Russia, the White Armies criss-crossed Central Asia. Tsydenov was committed to training practitioners who could endure life in such a world.

Foremost among his students were Dorje Badmaev, Tsydenov's main disciple, and Badmaev's stepson, Bidya Dandaron. In 1917, the Tsar was forced to abdicate, and soon Russia fell into utter chaos. The Cossack Army of Ataman Grigory Semyonov moved into Buryatia. Semyonov's troops, like all the armies of the time, lived by stealing from farmers, herdsmen, merchants, and peasants. This army was worse: they were murderers, rapists, and thieves. Semyonov finally was able to exert some discipline over his men, allied himself with Japanese troops near Manchuria, and took control of local governments through control of pre-existing dumas.

Under his rule, Mongolia, Siberia, and Buryatia established semi-autonomous domains. Nonetheless, in 1918 the Czech Legion was on the verge of taking control of the Trans-Siberian Railway. Baron Sternberg von Ungarn's army was moving to establish a Pan-Mongolian Empire. In the autumn, Semyonov decided to expand his forces by drafting young Buryat men.

It was at this point that Lubsan Samdan Tsydenov did something for which, if he is known at all, he is still remembered. All around him the world was collapsing into war as armies sought territory, wealth, and power. In the midst of this spreading violence and horror, he took advantage of both the Soviet proclamation of land reform, and the inability of the Red Army to move east. At the request of the Khori clan of the Buryats, some 13,000 families, Tsydenov assumed the role and title of Cakravartin, a Dharma King, proclaiming the establishment of a Buddhist kingdom, a realm that would exist entirely in accord with the Buddhist teachings. He said: "He who does not wish to fight, since fighting is contrary to the Buddha's law, let him come to me and be a subject in this kingdom."

He wrote:

"I really am a Dharma king of past, present, and future. This authority has been conferred on me by the spontaneous wisdom of the awakened state. It is my responsibility to save my subjects. We are bound together by the vow of nonviolence and by other vows to uphold the purity of life itself. Accordingly, no one may kill or serve in the army. There will be no army. Establishing this Buddhist state, I follow the principle of combining the religious and secular principles of government where authority is a union of those two. To rule is to accept the reality of life and death."

Tsydenov created a state modeled on both the rule of the Dalai Lama and on Western principles of elective democracy. All government positions, other than that of the Cakravartin ruler, were elected by secret ballot from among those who had been elected to the constituent assembly. He ordered a commission to create the government and other institutions of the new state, to be called Kudunai Erketei Balgasan, and its subjects were called Balagats. The immense faith and loyalty of Tsydenov's followers enabled his government to function simultaneously with that of Ataman Semyonov. Some citizens, even after the fall of the kingdom, continued to consider themselves subjects and practiced tantra as laypeople. All would be imprisoned or dead by 1935.

In early May of 1919, a week after this Buddhist state was formally established, agents of Semyonov's police arrested Tsydenov, along with nine members of his government. All were released once Tsydenov formally agreed to cooperate with Semyonov's government. This happened three more times in the same year. Each time, Tsydenov's release was taken as a sign of his magical invulnerability. Throughout the year, Tsydenov and his disciples taught, practiced, and administered his kingdom to the great contentment of his subjects. Even the death of his appointed successor, Badmaev, did not interrupt the progress of the kingdom. He appointed the five year old Dandaron to be his heir.

The ancestors have shown the unmistaken path.
Following them,
The Cakravartin's heart has broken open in the emptiness of space.

In the openness of the heart,
He dwells in the hidden expanse.

It was quite miraculous that, in such a tumultuous, hopeless, and violent climate, Tsydenov's Buddhist kingdom managed (by adhering to principles of non-violence) to flourish and protect tens of thousands of women, children, and men for more than a year. Even such a momentary achievement was still extraordinary. The Red Army, under General Tukhachevsky, began to overwhelm the various White Armies. Regional Bolshevik groups established local councils, ruling on behalf of the supreme Soviet. In May of 1920, Tsdenov was again arrested by Semyonov's agents and jailed in Verkhneudinsk. Six months later, Semyonov was driven from all the Buryat lands by the Red Army. Bolshevik forces gradually conquered the entire Russian Far East. So, by the end of 1920, the Red Army controlled all the territory of what had been Tsydenov's kingdom, and Tsydenov, still imprisoned in Verkhneudinsk, was now a captive of the Soviets. It was at that time he wrote a letter proclaiming the 7-year-old Dandaron would be his successor as Cakravartin.

In 1922, the Cheka (the Soviet secret police) moved Tsydenov 1400 miles from Verkhneudinsk to Novosibirsk. There he was isolated from contact with family, followers, or friends. He was not heard from again. According to an official statement, Tsydenov died in a military hospital in Novosibirsk on May 16, 1922. However, some said he was later taken to an unnamed labor camp farther north. In a third account, a man named Tsygan told V. Montlevich that in 1924 he had seen Tsydenov in the railway station in Verkhneudinsk. Tsydenov was dressed in an elegant European pin-striped suit. Tsygan greeted him and asked what he was doing. Tsydenov shook his hand and said that he was "going to Italy."

By the 1930s, all 44 Buddhist monasteries in Buryatia had been shut or destroyed. Their lamas — 15,000 to 17,000 of them — had been killed or imprisoned. Some 45,000 Buryats, considered rebels, had been murdered. Traditional Buryat culture was erased. Tsydenov's heir, Bidya Dandaron, spent the rest of his life in and out of forced labor camps in the Gulag system. It is said that throughout his imprisonment, he never stopped trying to find Tsydenov. He asked prisoners and prison guards if they had heard of him. Whether he knew his questions were in vain no one can say, but clearly Dandaron did not think that futility was a reason to stop searching. For the rest of the world, however, Tsydenov was a name written on some moldering files, recounted by aging storytellers in a string of curious episodes, images in a few grainy photographs, the name of one who was momentarily a protector, and, if fleetingly, a true Dharma King.

———A TELEPHONE CALL

It begins with a call from the doctor, and it is as I've often and unwillingly imagined: "I've got bad news."

There is a silent, airless implosion. I force myself to breathe, pull myself together, and ask whatever I can manage. The call ends, and I feel like the world is pulling away. I am being left behind. I put down the phone and make some notes about the disease, the treatments, the calls I'll need to make, then I burst into tears.

Outside the window there's a bright sunset and dark, pine-covered mountains. There's a cool evening breeze. How to tell my wife, my son, my family, my friends? I imagine how they are leading their lives assuming everything is going on as before. It's inconceivable that so much love, so much intensity, can just end. But a door has just closed. Everything in the world will vanish, and I will vanish. It may not be immediate, but it's now real. An innocuous little bump on my forehead has been diagnosed as nodular melanoma and mortality is no longer abstract. It's strange I feel so well.

There is, suddenly, an almost painful intensity to everything. I think of how Trungpa Rinpoche used the phrase "genuine mind of sadness" to point to an essential part of our lives. Sorrow, love, and being alive are inextricable.

The next days are taken up with trying to understand this form of cancer — its development, treatments, prognosis. My wife Debbie and I, always close, grow closer as we face a newly tenuous future. I tell my son and my good friends. Without being overly pessimistic or optimistic, I try to put them at ease. I try to continue with my normal activities, which now seem frail and contrived. More tests are scheduled, and visits to surgeons and oncologists are set up.

I think back to years ago when an acquaintance, Carlo, was dying of liver cancer. He wanted to go out with some guys, but not ones he'd been so very close to. Three of us went to a restaurant. Pasta with bottarga and all kinds of special dishes emerged; wine too. Carlo would suddenly be happy; then, in almost the same moment, he'd be desolate and heartbroken. He'd look away. Although my condition is nowhere near as grave as his, I realize how extraordinary was Carlo's willingness not to shrink from the overwhelming waves of love and sorrow.

As Naropa, the Indian mahasiddha, described it, living in conditioned existence is like "licking the honey on the razor's edge." Knowing we are close to the edge of it all, being lost brings to life a sudden intensity of love. Even if my mortality might be imminent, I'm overwhelmed with gratitude for everything that comes my way. Dare I say it, this disease has made me feel more alive.

I write to a friend who endured a long siege with lymphoma. He replies, "I certainly hope your 'mortality' is not that 'imminent.' But as you imply, it could be. To feel that is a great thing. I've always, always looked at my cancer as a great gift."

My sister-in-law enjoyed a long remission after grueling treatments for ovarian cancer. She was, as she acknowledged, utterly grateful for the transformation she experienced. She had no more time for the petty negativities that had previously undermined her. "I'll never regret it," she told me.

Relatives, friends, and acquaintances from all over begin to send me words of encouragement, prayers, and good wishes. Some I barely know: a local music critic, many friends of my wife's, members of her mother's church. The expanse of kindness is overwhelming and humbling. Many have been through similar experiences, and almost all know someone who has. What is happening to me is in no way unique.

When the test results indicate that my situation is rather less grave than it might have been, the congratulations from those around me convey a collective relief that I don't yet feel, though the warmth of everyone's embrace is palpable.

My surgery has been successful in removing all the melanoma that was detected. Nonetheless, I'm reluctant to view what I've been through as merely a scare or an unpleasant episode. I run into a friend who'd had a brain tumor. The surgery was risky, and many of the potential outcomes were terrifying. She tells me how, now that she's recovered, people want to say it's over and behind her. "I can't tell them," she admits, "but really, in a way, I don't even want it to be."

For me, a door has opened to living with less certainty, greater intensity, and far more gratitude. Fear of the cancer's return, future treatments, pain, and dying bring an enduring sharpness. Buddhist practice in this context is, as always, simply not getting caught in discursive elaborations.

Thoughts and feelings come and go. We do not choose what we think or feel. Love and friendship, the scent of the summer air, the shadows by the stream are each so uniquely valuable. So deeply to be loved. Everything seems new, bright, strangely exhilarating. It is, I feel shy to say, something like falling in love.

§ § §

A year or so later, I have lunch with my cousin Susan. She has weathered far greater medical trials than this. A lot of what she went through was so long ago that she no longer feels the same intensity of gratitude.

This may be so, but I hope she won't mind if I say that I feel in her a depth of strength, humor, warmth, and vivacity that is greater than before. One does not, I think, encounter one's mortality without something new emerging, and it is not just one thing.

Around the same time, I felt decisively that I was entering into old age. It was different than anything I had assumed. My son (29 years old at the time) said to me: "You're only as old as you think you are."

"Only young people think that," I found myself snapping.

Nonetheless, it has become evident that people resent acknowledging sickness, aging, and the evidence of mortality in others. They are actually quite aggressive about it. Reflecting on this led me, by not the most direct of routes, to considering how a Prince who lived in sequestered luxury was shocked to discover the universality of old age, sickness, and death. These shocks then led this Prince directly to becoming the Buddha and opening a new path of liberation in the world. The following four pieces are explorations of those discoveries.

FOUR DIVINE MESSENGERS:

1 — ENCOUNTERING OLD AGE

It is said that we who live within the mists do not see the shapes of the clouds that are our dwelling place. We do not see the radiance of the sun, the moon, the stars, nor do we know the vastness of the sky.

There are many stories of children, young men and young women, princesses and princes, whose parents determined to shield them from suffering and obstacles. They were raised behind high castle walls. There are many stories of men and women who never dared to leave the security of their palaces, but could not silence the whispers of the high winds or avoid fugitive and nameless fears.

An old man in the elevator is shaking his head. In a bitter voice he tells me how sick he has been, that aging "takes so much away from you. You lose so much."

I am in the same situation, of course, and feel resistant to his depression. I wonder. Isn't there more to it? Suddenly I want to know: "But what does old age give?"

It is said that more than two thousand years ago in the north of India, there was a Prince, Siddhartha, who lived in a palace amid flower gardens filled with the sounds of bells, music, fountains, and songbirds. The King, his father, made sure he was surrounded by strong and lively young men, and beautiful, sensitive women. The king determined that his son would train to succeed him, without ever knowing fear, suffering, or sadness.

And yet the Prince was curious. One day, he ordered his charioteer to take him in his golden chariot to explore the world outside the palace gates. He passed through the bustling crowds that filled the boulevards and marketplaces of his father's capitol. Lingering at the edges of a crowd was a couple, a woman and a man, both bent over, gaunt, tremulous, worn out. Their veins stood out on their bodies, their teeth chattered, and their desiccated skin was a maze of cracks and wrinkles. They turned their heads anxiously in all directions, for they could not see well. People bumped into them, for they could not hear. Gray hairs hung from their scalps; their eyelids had no lashes, and were crusty and red-rimmed. Their heads wavered, and their hands shook. They had the sour smell of decay. The Prince asked his charioteer:"What are these? Has nature made them thus, or is it chance?"

The charioteer answered: "Sire, these creatures are like all others who live into the twilight of their years. They are merely old. They were once children nursing at their mother's breast; they grew, they were young, they had strength and beauty and they were brave, enterprising, lustful; they married, they raised their families, their lives were full. Now they are near the end of life. They suffer from the press of time that mars beauty, ruins vigor, kills pleasure, weakens memory, destroys the senses. Old age has seized these men and broken them. It has taken away all their friends and people they could rely on. They are like an abandoned house on an island amid a torrential flood. They are the ruin of what once they were."

The Prince asked: "Will this also be my fate?"

The charioteer replied: "My lord, no one who lives can escape this."

The Prince shuddered like a bull at the sound of thunder. He uttered a deep sigh and shook his head. His eyes wandered from the wretched men to the happy crowds. "The world is not frantic with terror! How can they ignore our common fate?"

This was Prince Siddhartha's first meeting with old age. For an instant, the Prince saw through the surface of his existence as if seeing through a painted screen. Meeting old age, he encountered the first of the Divine Messengers. It was his first glimpse of the truth. Terror, sorrow, the hope to escape — all are irrelevant.

Tinnitus, less energy, a slightly less reliable faculty of recall, various incapacities — these are signs of aging, but I do not feel the process of getting old. In the mirror is a man, almost a stranger, 70 years old. But my mind, my habits of mind, the ways in which I am accustomed to thinking and feeling, the ways I expected myself to be, have not much changed. The feeling of being old comes in sudden flashes.

The doctor diagnoses a nodular melanoma. Excised, it leaves an interesting scar. Statistics indicate a truncated life expectancy. I feel the same as before, and I do not. Information has changed me as much as any virus or germ. It tells me I am moving into terrains that are uncontrollable, unknowable.

A renowned specialist has nothing of use for me. "Is there any other way I can help?" he asks. I smile. "If you can tell me the two things I doubt you know." He raises his eyebrows. "How long will I last, and how bad will it hurt?" He gives a rueful shrug.

I feel the world slightly moving away. I am not different, really. Or the way in which I sense myself as different is difficult to grasp. But I do know that my body and world are changing in unexpected ways. I am being separated from a life I know. A new world presents itself, sharp, vivid, uncompromising. It is not what I expected.

I watch young women and men, full of certainty that the intensity of their desires, the anarchic power of appetites, the bright newness of their thoughts and insights, will surely make the world bend before them. With the sheer intensity of their sexual desire, of wanting and longing; how could they think otherwise?

Living on the edge of uncertainty is somehow stimulating. The world is opening beneath my feet.

It is said that the awakened state is the natural state. It is said that the awakened state is all-pervasive as space.

It is said that there are more Buddhas, Buddha realms, kinds of teachings, realizations, assemblies of beings sharing those teachings than there are grains of sand in the Ganges and in all the beds of all the seas, combined with all the universes of galaxies of stars.

It is said that every instant in the flow of illusion and suffering displays the full panoply of the unimpeded awakened state. There are no moments in which awake is not.

The core of the feeling that plagues us is that we are missing something.

I am changing in ways that are both visible and utterly unfamiliar. And I am as I always was. I am missing something.

It is a time of sudden vast surprise.

My friend's father was a big man, even in his late 90s. His hands were huge and strong. He had been a warehouse foreman and spent most of his life in the Bronx. He loved New York, and, finding himself now at the end of his life, living with his son in a suburban house with a tree-filled backyard, he was occasionally disoriented. It didn't really make sense that he would end up in such a place.

He often sat in the yard, amid the trees. "It's amazing," he said, "I had no idea that there were so many kinds of green."

The world we know is aging and dying, falling beneath the hordes of the new.

What inspired us, what drew us on, the prospect of making something new in the world, some kind of new home, new love, new child, the prospect of living, all this is being worn out. The house is old, the lover has gotten sick, the children are adults and have their concerns. And the sense of what was valuable, important, necessary to promulgate, these are values no longer so widely shared. Perhaps in earlier times there were values that transcended generational limits, now they barely survive a single human life.

The world we have worked for is neither fresh nor (to those younger than us) desirable.

"You're only as old as you think you are," my son says.

"Oh, only young people think that," I say.

The world is aging, dying.

We look at those we love. We look at those whose intimacy sustains us. Their bodies are betraying them. They are in decline. Their minds are in retreat. They look at us tenderly, but their glance moves inward to secret fears and losses of their own. Among these losses, they are looking at us, our bodies, our minds in retreat from a world that is losing us.

The younger, as they must and should, struggle to grasp and hold on. They look at us and turn away. The vector of our existence is not the same as theirs. It is the time of parting.

Unexpected perspectives appear, new light shines on enduring patterns and new intensities. More than ever before we are faced with utter uncertainty. More even than when we were adolescents, we are moving into something completely unknown. It is frightening, and so very interesting, seductive even.

Memory no longer chained to the pragmatics of seizing and holding.

We are dazzled among patterns. We now enter a world and worlds transforming unimaginably. We are being changed without regard to pain or dignity or accomplishment or punishment or regret. Even the forms of consciousness that we believe are valuable or true will not necessarily sustain us. Uncertainty is unceasing.

The past becomes vivid and slippery.

I am looking across the front seat of the speeding car at my grandfather. He is looking intently through his pince-nez glasses at the black-top rippling in the summer air. He looks over at me, and I look away. The cicadas are churning the air. I am eight years old.

The spotlight reflected off the green-robed tenor's naked sword flashes suddenly across the vast auditorium, right into my eyes. I am eleven years old. He turns and begins to sing. Why do such moments come unbidden? Why are they now so clear?

Memories no longer quite provide the story of why things are the way they are. They arise as the framework that once linked them seems to fall out from underneath. I have far less to hide. I am suddenly and shamefully aware of specific moments when I have disappointed parents, teachers, friends, lovers, strangers, my son, my wife. I cringe, but there is nothing to be done.

Moments as a baby, child, adolescent, young and then older man, loom vivid and clear. Moments, once markers of some effortful identity, each with different tonalities, thrusts, senses of containment, now display new patterns as former meanings drift.

I am looking out the window of a train as day turns to night, as landscapes unfold, become briefly more intense, and the train hurtles toward a sunset I cannot see.

And I recall driving east over a ridge into Arizona at sunset. A great basin already in shadow opens as far as the eye can see. Far to the north, a mysterious array of mesas and buttes glow in the orange light while beyond, a dark red palisade blocks the horizon. These huge formations seem to flow across the tawny desert floor like a secret epic now being enacted just beneath the threshold of thought and memory.

Late in life, many artists have painted, written, and composed work that is far different from what they had done earlier, and far different from work anyone else had done. The late works of Bach, Michelangelo, Titian, Beethoven, Stravinsky, and Matisse (to mention a few) expand on what they did before, but enter unexpected new terrain. This work often is a summit that does not illuminate the past nor provide a pathway to any known future.

To begin the dance theater of Japan, Hata came from Korea. He said:

Theater is the genius of the old.
The world draws way from them;
Their horizon widens.
The wide world is seen for what it is.
It draws away.
The future shortens
And the past speaks with greater clarity.

The body is no longer the focus of the world.
Beings of light show themselves.

Driving on a gray dirt road, scraggly yellow sunflowers on either side. It's late morning. The sun is pale and the dusty soil pale gray. I'm a little lost. The road occasionally runs through a stand of skinny leafless trees. It's a cool day in mid-spring. I'm looking for a crossroads that will get me back to... that leads to another road that will take me wherever it is I'm going.

I am sleeping, dreaming. But is this a dream? As I dream, it seems slightly familiar, but I can't remember anything like this in waking life. I wonder. Perhaps this is a return in dream to a dream landscape that occasionally appears. It is not a particularly meaningful place. Pale, gray, gritty soil, and pale blue sky, bright yellow flowers, and being lost here, but not seriously so. I'm quite certain that I'll find the way to wherever it was I was intending to go.

But I know I'm dreaming, and I want to remember this. I am wondering if this is just some landscape hovering in space to which I have inadvertently returned. A set of images through which a mind that is mine, for no reason, is just passing through.

I wake and work to remember. Yes, it is a real place, a place near Salida, Colorado. I was driving there with my wife. We were momentarily and pleasantly lost on the way home. It is ordinary and strange.

Mrs. T. was not like any of my mother's friends. Witty, dark and sensuous, she held herself with mysterious reserve. Eyes wide open, smile amused, a bit aloof, she favored both the men who flirted and the women who whispered as she entered the room with ironic merriment. She was wickedly good at card games, too. Of course, she'd had a discreet face-lift. She'd been widowed twice before she was 28.

We wrote to each other at Christmas. She was in her mid-90s, living in a nursing home. Her correspondence had become less and less detailed. I did not know whom to ask about her condition. Finally my card was returned, stamped DECEASED.

The year before, she had written only: "You know, I'm very flattered that you think I'm still within reach of the US Postal Service."

FOUR DIVINE MESSENGERS:

2 — SICKNESS

I dream I am descending in an old oak-paneled elevator. Suddenly I am aware of someone behind me. Tensing, I turn. A wild elfin man in a tweed suit with wild orange hair, a face like Mr. Punch, is leering at me. I am terrified, powerless to move or cry out. My heart stops. I panic. Suddenly I wake, very weak, covered in sweat, still unable to move.

Bright sunlight blurs on the edges of the window. Warm white sheets are absorbing me.

When Prince Siddhartha returned to his palace after seeing the sorrows of old age, for many weeks he could find no peace or pleasure. Eventually he returned to the pastimes of a Prince, and became again engulfed in studies, swordplay, and luxury. But his curiosity again returned, and he decided once more to ride in his chariot through the city.

As Siddhartha rode past a shouting and laughing crowd, one man staggered from the bushes and fell on the road before his chariot. People looked at the man, but quickly moved away. No one would help him. Siddhartha asked the charioteer: "Why is this man lying there shivering but covered with sweat, with a distended belly but withered arms, pale as ash, white spit dried around his lips and moaning in agony, crying for water? He gasps for breath. But those walking past avert their gaze and shun him. Charioteer, what is this man?"

The charioteer answered: "My lord, this man is sick. Disease has ravaged his body. He is weak; yet he, too, was once healthy and strong! People avoid him lest they too catch his illness."

The Prince looked at the man with pity, and asked again: "Is this affliction peculiar to this man, or are all creatures threatened with sickness?"

He answered: "We, too, will all suffer from some such affliction. O Prince, sickness prowls constantly through the world. It feeds on everything alive, and cannot be escaped."

When the Prince heard this painful truth, he began to tremble like a moonbeam reflected in the waves of the sea, and he uttered these words of bitterness and pity: "Men see suffering and sickness, yet they never lose their self-confidence! Oh, how great must be their ignorance! They are constantly threatened with disease, yet they can still laugh and be merry! Turn your horses around. Our pleasure trip has ended. Let us return to the palace. I have learned to fear sickness. My soul turns away from the world. Like a flower deprived of light, it is withering."

From time to time, and for no known reason, approximately 200 different kinds of cells, each with as many as 20 sub-groups, coalesce in a complex dance. Coming together and dissipating at varying rates, replacing themselves, or not, they move through time and space, adopting momentary configurations, in gestures of complexity, power, and grace. Just like the galaxies that take shape on a much vaster scale of space and time, the purpose or meaning of these temporary configurations are subjects of constant speculation, terror, belief, legend, dream, and myth.

Names have been given to each cell according to the functions which humans value. There are surely many other kinds of cells in these configurations, but their functions are neither valued nor known. Here, by name:

Exocrine secretory epithelial, hormone secreting, keratinizing epithelial, wet stratified barrier epithelial, sensory transducer, autonomic neuron, sense organ and peripheral neuron supporting, central nervous system neurons and glial, lens, derived primarily from mesoderm, metabolism and storage, barrier functions (lung, gut, exocrine glands and urogenital tract), kidney, extragular matrix, contractile, blood and immune systems, germs, nurse, interstitials, exocrine secretory epithelial, mucous including fructose for swimming sperm, prostate gland, bulbourethral gland, Bartholin's gland, gland of Littre, uterus endometrium, isolated goblet of respiratory and digestive tracts, stomach lining mucous gastric chief, panethal of small intestine, type II pneumocyte of lung, clara of lung, hormone secreting, anterior pituitary, somatotropes lactotropes, thyrotropes, gonadotropes, corticotropes, intermediate pituitary, secreting melanocyte-stimulating hormone, magnocellular neurosecretory cells, secreting oxytocin, secreting vasopressin, gut and respiratory tract, secreting serotonin, secreting endorphin, secreting somatostatin, secreting gastrin, secreting secretin, secreting cholecystokinin, secreting insulin, secreting glucagon, secreting bombesin, thyroid gland, thyroid epithelial parafollicular, parathyroid gland, parathyroid chief oxyphil, adrenal glands, secreting corticosteroids, Leydig, theca interna, corpus luteum, granita lutein, luteins, juxtaglomerular, macula densa, peripolar, mesangial, integumentary system, keratinizing epithelial, epidermal keratinocyte, epidermal basal, keratinocyte of fingernails and toenails, nail bed basal, medullary hair shaft, cortical hair shaft, cuticular hair shaft, cuticular hair root sheath, hair root sheath of Huxley's layer, hair root sheath of Henle's layer, external hair root sheath, hair matrix, wet stratified barrier epithelial, surface epithelial of stratified squamous, basal of epithelia of cornea, tongue, oral cavity, esophagus, anal canal, distal urethra and vagina, urinary epithelium. There are nerves, also known as neurons, present in our human body. They are branched out. These make up nervous tissue. A neuron consists of a body with a nucleus and cytoplasm, from which long thin hair-like parts arise. Sensory transducers, auditory inner hair of organ of Corti, auditory outer hair of organ of Corti, basal of olfactory epithelium, cold-sensitive primary sensory neurons, heat-sensitive primary sensory neurons, Merkel of epidermis, olfactory receptor neuron, pain-sensitive primary sensory neurons, photoreceptor rods, photoreceptor blue-sensitive cone of eye, photoreceptor green-sensitive cone of eye, photoreceptor red-sensitive cone of eye, proprioceptive primary sensory neurons (various types), touch-sensitive primary sensory neurons (various types), type I carotid body (blood pH sensor), type II carotid body (blood pH sensor), type I hair of vestibular system of ear (acceleration and gravity), type II hair of vestibular system of ear (acceleration and gravity), autonomic neuron, cholinergic neural (various types), adrenergic neural (various types), peptidergic neural, inner pillar of organ of Corti, outer pillar of organ of Corti, inner phalangeal of organ of Corti, outer phalangeal of organ of Corti, border of organ of Corti, Hensen of organ of Corti, vestibular apparatus supporting, taste bud supporting, olfactory epithelium supporting, Schwann, satellite glial (encapsulating peripheral nerve bodies), enteric glial, central nervous system neurons and glials, astrocyte (various types), neuron (large variety of types, still poorly classified), oligodendrocyte, spindle neuron, crystallin, derived primarily from mesoderm [metabolism and storages,] hepatocyte, adipocytes, white fat, brown fat, liver lipocyte, barrier functions (lung, gut, exocrine glands and urogenital tract), kidney parietal, kidney glomerulus podocyte, kidney proximal tubule brush border, loop of Henle thin segment, kidney distal tubule, kidney collecting duct, type I pneumocyte (lining air space of lung), pancreatic duct (centroacinar), non-striated duct (of sweat gland, salivary gland, mammary gland, etc.), principal, intercalated, duct (of seminal vesicle, prostate gland, etc.), intestinal brush border (with microvilli), exocrine gland striated duct, gall bladder epithelial, ductulus efferens nonciliated, epididymal principal, epididymal basal, extracellular matrices, ameloblast epithelial (tooth enamel secretion), planum semilunatum epithelial of vestibular system of ear (proteoglycan secretion), organ of Corti interdental epithelial (secreting tectorial membrane-covering hairs), loose connective tissue fibroblasts, corneal fibroblasts (corneal keratocytes), tendon fibroblasts, bone marrow reticular tissue fibroblasts, other non-epithelial fibroblasts, pericyte, nucleus pulposus of intervertebral disc, cementoblast/cementocyte (tooth root bonelike ewan secretion), odontoblast/odontocete (tooth dentin secretion), hyaline cartilage chondrocyte, fibrocartilage chondrocyte, elastic cartilage chondrocyte, osteoblast/osteocyte, osteoprogenitor (stem of osteoblasts), hyalocyte of vitreous body of eye, stellate of perilymphatic space of ear, hepatic stellate (ito), pancreatic stelle, contractile, skeletal muscle, red skeletal muscle (slow), white skeletal muscle (fast), intermediate skeletal muscle, nuclear bag of muscle spindle, nuclear chain of muscle spindle, satellite, ordinary heart muscle, nodal heart muscle, Purkinje fiber, smooth muscle, myoepithelial of iris, myoepithelial of exocrine glands, erythrocyte, megakaryocyte, monocyte, connective tissue macrophage, epidermal Langerhans, osteoclast, dendritic, microglial, neutrophil granulocyte, eosinophil granulocyte, basophil granulocyte, hybridoma, mast, helper T, suppressor T, cytotoxic T, natural killer T and B, natural killer, reticulocyte, stems and committed progenitors for the blood and immune system, germ, oogonium/oocyte, spermatid, spermatocyte, spermatogonium, spermatozoon, nurse, ovarian follicle, sertoli, interstitials [interstitial kidneys].

The cell types emerge, proliferate, decay at varying rates, are replaced or not. They dissolve back into space and emerge in new forms. 37.5 trillion such cells call out, draw together, bind, release, expand, and contract in a pattern known as a person.

They assemble. They dance, re-assemble, continue. Elements spin away; some exhaust themselves, wear out. Some are replaced and continue. Trillions upon trillions of different cells, drifting in empty space, are coalescing as colonies, are swaying, dissolving, reforming, continuing, even as mysterious clouds of viral colonies, known or unknown to each other, are on the move. These have no memory of continuing, only the fact of continuing.

As tribes of humankind multiply, migrate, and take possession of the earth, all for reasons they themselves do not know, viral colonies stir. They are dislodged when the permafrost beneath a campfire thaws. They move when a bird eats a spider in the high forest. The bird is shot, cooked on the fire, eaten. The shamans of the north have seen these minute beings on the move. They pass through denser forms of space in soil, pond waters, flesh. They sense themselves only as a cloud taking shape within other forms. They change the lives of those they inhabit. They change the actions of cells dancing in the shape of skin, brain, blood, and inner organs. They change our experience of mind and world.

A friend woke up feeling strangely apprehensive and, within a very short period of time, he found himself completely paralyzed. His nerves were on fire. Doctors had a name for what was happening, but no way to resolve it. The pain, his terror, and claustrophobia cannot be imagined. He thought of his teacher constantly. He found that when he let himself dissolve a sense of boundary between himself and the totality of his situation, the intensity eased. He felt the boundaries of the body in which he was trapped open into an immense expanse. There he rested until a flickering thought reintroduced the specifics of imprisonment. It was a path of surrender, repeated, of necessity, endlessly and over a few years it led back to speech and mobility.

In the life of persons, patterns intersect with other kinds of patterns, and this dance changes both. The interaction causes elements in the pattern that is a woman or man or child or elder to sicken. They weaken as organs fail, and the larger pattern moves towards incoherence. Experienced as fever, as cold, as dementia, paralysis, impairments and pain of all kinds, it is sickness.

Now the body can no longer be taken for granted. Awareness encounters sharp obstacles moving on the body's recently complaisant streams. Suddenly actions, responses, and simple continuing do not take place with ease or certainty. Breathing, swallowing, ingestion, excretion, standing, sitting, walking, sleeping, and waking do not happen without pain or difficulty. The medical procedures inflicted to make them possible are painful and humiliating. The body is no longer a location of strength and pleasure. Patterns of expectation are wrenched out of shape. The body becomes a location of pain and faint disgust, the senses are corrupted. Smell and taste carry a slight aura of rot or of chemical overlay.

The sick are living in their bodies like people trapped in a war-ravaged city. All of daily life is uncertain, difficult, filled with threats of death and dismemberment. That life continues is an act of inexplicable will or mindless desperation. They scurry through the dust-filled air, dodging amongst the fragments of life. Those with weapons fire into the smoke and shadows. All others flee, struggling through the rubble of once-familiar avenues to find the means to continue living and knowing, all the while that there is no hope of escape.

From time to time, the gunfire, the explosions, the shouting suddenly stop. Hiding in the shadow of a cellar wall, a child looks up. The sky is clear, still blue. It is incomprehensible.

Peter once said: "In my obituary, don't let anyone say I battled cancer. I was a battleground."

The link that binds the senses to the past and establishes the thrust of continuing is suddenly fraying. A splitting headache, an uncontrollable tremor, a cramp, sudden loss of balance, a growing tentativeness altogether take hold. The linkages themselves are vibrating on their own. White rainbows swirl around the circle at the edge of sight.

He feels his atoms flying apart in all directions. The center is uncertain. The inner network, the outer skin, the conceptual web of agreed upon realities, all are stretched. He feels an indifferent vast emptiness encompassing him. Inexplicable dream states emerge from nowhere. Visions come to life and linger like dreams on waking. Everything that seemed solid is wavering and porous.

She had a chest cold for ten days. Sickness swept her into a flow she could not get out of. She was being drawn away from the world. She was shifting into a separate time stream. She was immersed in a body-stream now going its own way. She was carried onto a subterranean river, drawn through caverns and passages, and could not stop.

She thought she might be close to death. She felt that she was someone that existed only in her memory. She was aware how thin the membrane was that bound her to life. The membrane was stretching. In the moments when the fear abates, it is, in a way, interesting.

Artur Lundquist lived through WWII, which marked him deeply. At seventy-five he had a stroke, and lay in a coma for two months. From the time he woke, his recovery was slow but filled with dreams and imaginings. He wrote an account of what he experienced:

> "Stranger within me, stranger at my side. I live in several eras flowing in different directions…how easy to lift past the surface and perceive its strange reality… as the present falls endlessly backwards and rises again in front of us, is born and dies in the same moment to gather at the river which flows slowly at the same time beyond us and before us."

Timeless: whatever conventions require or intentions demand, these no longer have any traction on the surface of a time now defined by the body's pain, the mind's anguish. The body is being transformed. The agents of change are not part of our desire or understanding. We are being deformed, submerged in flesh that is burning or cold, flaccid or in spasm. Our awareness is now deeper within this flesh, the movement of fluids and solids. The outer world is relevant only as a support to continuing or ending, only as offering ease or greater pain. He was falling through the network of needs that had kept him in the human world. His body was a vessel of skin and bone floating on the dark hot water of the Styx. And who was the pilot? It was no longer he. He had pushed off from the bank where others called to him, and he soundlessly called back to them.

He recoiled from the pain in his chest. His awareness shrank within the body. His mind moved in this inner space and seemed to sense barely perceptible worlds, entering them, becoming them, moving.

Illness, fever, and pain determined when he woke and slept. They prompted the dreams which, even when unconscious, he recognized were not quite his own. At times he floated in a silent space, empty, cool, and motionless.

My friend Tom had a stroke. He found himself imprisoned in his mind. He was unable to speak. He knew the words and how to order them. He had forgotten nothing. But his body, and all the physical world, had become hard, bright, and solid. He was encased in a seamless continuum of things. Words, thoughts, feelings could not be inserted anywhere between them.

A bank of purple clouds
Against the pale blue-gray above the mountains
Darker with feathered borders descending
Perhaps rain is to come,
Perhaps it is falling deep in the mountains.

moment

In its own frame of reference.

Not ours,
Its sky mind
Does not answer our questions
Or speak in our solitude.

Its cloud thought
Does not articulate
Need or time

moment

The lover turns her back.
Her long beautiful spine,
Pale soft skin.
She puts on her robe
And leaves the room.

moment

I dreamed I ...

I am hurtling through dimensions I cannot comprehend. I am burnt and frozen, squeezed, distended. Things are pushed into being and pulled out. And there's no stopping, no stopping of the intensity, the claustrophobia, pain, and the intermittent brightness of a shimmering vast expanse.

Gap

On and on, forgetting and now remembering that moment when you first came up the escalator in a red dress. Such beauty, such terror, such intensity, such expanses of dissolving boundaries. I am being devoured. I am in a whirlwind. I will not emerge as the one I once knew.

Gap

A recurring dream makes an appearance. Late at night I am walking home alone on the shabby part of a main thoroughfare, dimly lit with brownish yellow sodium streetlights. At first it is a familiar part of the city where I lived for many years. The boulevard has a slightly upward incline lined with old movie theaters, Chinese and Cuban restaurants, cheap clothes stores.

I feel a sudden urgency to find something to take home to eat. I enter a dark narrow specialty food shop with a high ceiling. The refrigerator cabinets are lit by bluish fluorescent lights. I am walking along, trying to see what is in the coolers, trying to make a choice. Cheeses, tin foil containers of lasagna, frozen beef stew, guava paste. Nothing looks appealing enough. Moving deeper into the store, there are racks upon racks of tired once-trendy clothes on either side. I am curious, but don't want to take the time to stop.

I am alone. I keep moving. Nothing is bright or fresh or vivid. Nothing looks the way it might once have. There are no other customers, no salespeople, no one else walking home.

FOUR DIVINE MESSENGERS:

3 — DEATH

In his 80s, the great Zen master Kyozan Joshu Sasaki Roshi was ill and in the hospital, but hearing that one of his earliest Western students was dying, he left and took an airplane across the country to see her.

"Roshi, I'm so afraid of dying," she said. He moved very close to her.

"That's irrelevant now," he whispered.

She nodded.

Beneath endless blue skies, hidden in recesses of the vast steppes' rolling plains, stand the Cities of the Dead. Near small lakes and streams, but far from any roads, stand dozens of walled cities with their silent occupants. Their gates are open, but limestone walls surround the ornate buildings crowded within. Above the carved stonework float turquoise domes and sharp gold minarets. The facades are decorated with stone galleries and painted murals of the stern-faced occupants in their white turbans and long red robes. Other mausoleums are decorated with copper intaglios of the deceased. Bronze statues of angels and rearing horses surmount pointed towers. Craftsmen from afar come to build these structures. The deceased are installed with lavish feasts and ceremonies. Afterwards, the living do not visit here. They do not interfere with the ways of the dead, nor bother them in their new abodes. They allow the buildings to crumble, and the occupants to return to the earth.

Travelers who chance to come upon these cities see them sparkling in the distance and are drawn by their splendor. They find, as they come closer, the cities diminish in size, and when they stand at the cities' gates, they cannot enter. No matter how small the living visitors may be, they are much too large.

In the Tibetan text called *The Bardo Thodol* or *Liberation Through Hearing*, it is said that at certain points between death and rebirth, our consciousness is overwhelmed by the all-encompassing brilliance of the wakened state. Simultaneously, we become aware of more comfortable, more pleasant, and familiar shades of muted lights nearby. The text urges us to avoid these, and to surrender into the vast and uncompromising brilliance of what is actually our own mind.

§ § §

Now Prince Siddhartha again returned to his former princely preoccupations, but he could not so easily forget that he had seen that all are fated to endure old age and sickness. Again he grew restless and ill at ease. He wanted to know more of the fate of those who live in this world. He summoned his chariot and once more set forth.

This time he saw a procession of men and women weeping. On their shoulders they carried a stretcher. On it was the form of a woman wrapped in cotton, shrunken, brittle, motionless. Her face was gray, her mouth open, but she did not breathe. Flies crawled in and out of her nose, but she did not react. She was rigid and lifeless as a stick of dried wood. Those carrying her, and all those in the procession, were weeping and crying.

The Prince asked: "What is that thing in the shape of a deformed woman? It is rigid and immobile, and must be carried by others. It is followed by a small crowd wailing and wearing white clothes. What is this being? She does not seem to suffer. What is she doing?"

The charioteer replied: "My Lord, she has neither intelligence nor feeling nor breath. She sleeps without consciousness, like grass or a piece of wood. She is insensitive to pleasure or suffering. Friends, family, enemies — all have no meaning for her. Her consciousness no longer animates her body. Sire, she is dead."

The Prince was troubled. He said: "Is this woman the only one stricken in this way?"

The charioteer answered: "No. This is the end that awaits every living being. Death consumes all that lives. What is left is a husk, a shell that has no consciousness."

The Prince was disturbed. He asked: "And where has it gone, this life, this consciousness?"

"No one knows, my Lord. But certainly many religions and many philosophies have taught that a soul or consciousness has an afterlife."

"Is this true?"

"All we know are visions and words from living men and women. The dead do not speak."

Prince Siddhartha reflected for a long time. He listened to the wind fluttering in the palms; he smelled smoke from cook fires; he saw women in their silk robes walking in a park, and heard children shouting happily.

"So we know we will die, but we do not know anything beyond that?"

"Death, my Lord, is the end of our understanding."

Then Prince Siddhartha knew what death was. He shuddered and leaned against the chariot. His words were full of distress and amazement: "And we cannot stop it. Our minds teem with theories. We struggle and we kill to take control of destiny. We fill the world with dreams. No matter, we will die. No matter, we do not know when or why or for what purpose."

The charioteer did not answer, and they returned to the palace in silence. Passing through the villages and forests, passing by men herding cattle, women carrying baskets, seeing that some were happy, others sad, and knowing none, not one, would leave a trace upon the earth, a vast sorrow and estrangement encompassed him.

Why not imagine that, if there is continuing, it is like the wind. It rises and falls and rises and is never the same. It rises and falls and swirls and stops, and out of nowhere is gentle, and out of nowhere is violent and vengeful. Continuing, it destroys and creates and goes everywhere around the globe. It continues through the night of space, sliding under window sills and on. And does this wind refer to any single moment in its moving as defining itself? As establishing the way in which it is?

In what way does the wind know itself, or what it has touched, or any of its other experiences? In its continuing and stopping and continuing, in the circumstances from which it arises, in the situations it nurtures, caresses, animates, destroys, it does not refer to past or future, knowing or not knowing, consciousness or utter absence of consciousness.

Shall we call such wind Buddha Nature? Shall we call such continuing Buddha Nature?

I was three years old, and I lay on the dining room floor in the mid-morning sun. I pretended I was dead and did not move. I felt the bright heat of the sun pass through me and into the soft green and red weaving of the old oriental rug. I heard voices in the kitchen. I did not move. Yesterday, I was standing in the front yard looking up at towers of white clouds in the deep blue sky. Could something live there? A squeal of car brakes, then an animal screamed. A robin's egg blue car pulled to the curb. Our dog lay writhing on the pavement in front of it. A small man in short sleeves stood anxiously nearby. She did not die immediately, and I watched as her legs trembled and her eyes spun around in every direction.

Like her, I now bared my teeth and opened my eyes. Dust motes sparkled in the air like a million alien worlds.

I sat in a movie theater between the woman who would soon be my wife and the man who was my close friend and later collaborator on several large theater pieces. We were watching a horror movie, and the scene, which was not particularly scary, took place in a surgical operating room. Suddenly the screen was suffused with an intense fluorescent green-white light.

This light, it seemed, poured through my body and between my cells. It felt like I was coming apart. Suddenly there was a violent pain in my chest. My heart felt like a clenched fist, and stopped beating. I moved my ribs side to side, up and down, to loosen the contraction in my chest. I could barely breathe.

At first, I panicked; then I watched. I knew I could let go. The light was there, cold and pale, and I could slide along it. Simultaneously, I felt that I still had more to do. My fate with my wife-to-be and my friend was not yet complete. I had to get away from the light. My heart hurt terribly. I forced myself up, stumbled into the aisle, and fell, cutting my head. People laughed. I picked myself up and crashed through the doors and foyer onto the street. I sat on the curb and covered my eyes.

The man and woman took me home. I went to bed, and for the next day wore dark glasses and kept the shades drawn. Anything, it seemed, but the dimmest light could end my life.

Death, no one can come to terms with it.

We can no more come to terms with it than we can with living. We know our life will end, and we tell a story of a character who starts, acts, ends. But we ourselves do not know our own beginning; the middle is uncertain and without shape; the end is a horizon with no sky beyond.

Yes. We invent things. We can say the essence, the soul, will live forever. We say this invisible part of the dead person, this memory really, is on its own journey. We say this because we think we are on a journey, moving on. We say that after death the soul of the deceased is judged. We say this because we the living are still judging them.

But suddenly someone you know, a part of your world, is not there. There is a gap.

And there is a corpse smelling sour and rotting. Gray, yellow, chalky, green, bloodless. It is disposed of. Then, day after day, like a scab forming, the world reforms with a scar, rippled and more brittle, then fading. We cannot come to terms with it. We can only continue.

A doctor tells you that the little pain you have is an illness that will kill you. He does not know when. There is a sudden wave of great sadness knowing now you will be parted from all else, everything you love and know. Feeling expands to the breadth of the sky. A friend says: "Love never dies." But there is the sorrow of not comprehending, not fully appreciating, and how things end always incomplete. There is eating and shitting and fucking and sleeping and working. There are moments of accomplishment and failure. There is leaving a mark and forgetting where it was. There is the haunted sorrow of incompleteness, the fragmented.

And, slowly, a subtle and illicit allure of coming to an end now comes insidiously to us.

The sun warms and burns us. The wind presses and chills. The snow makes the world still and beautiful. The moon waxes and wanes, drawing sea tides and blood. The soil upholds us and nourishes us, and takes our bodies back into itself. And in the night we see the stars, constellations hinting at meanings, their slow traversals implying vaster scales of time.

In darkness, we imagine. Our minds do not cease imagining good and evil, structures that will endure, true pathways and consolations that will never fail. Our minds give impetuous existence to gods and goddesses, to hopes that the world and we are continuing. The stars hint at terms of reference. Our impending death pushes us on to search for coming to terms.

The visitors pass along a road, finding themselves between a green stagnant pond and an enclosed complex of temples and outbuildings, all painted in violent crimson. The walls, the towers, the roof, all are painted the color of fresh blood. This, they are told, is the House of Kali. It is a place of sacrifice and worship, her shrine, her temple, her abode.

Their guide tells them: her name means destruction, her name means death, her name means time. She is the great wrathful mother, the destroyer and origin of all. Her naked black body is covered with blood that pours from her mouth as she consumes the universe. She wears a necklace of skulls, and lightning flashes in her hair. Her three bloodshot eyes are past, present, and future. She smells of blood and semen, feces, urine, and burning flesh. Her voice combines silence and thunder.

They hear people inside the walls chanting to invoke the goddess:

HUM HUM HUM

Surrounded by twisting clouds of oily black smoke
Choking all of space,
Surrounded by shooting sparks of exploding suns, moons on fire,
Galaxies being ripped apart,
Seated on a throne of fire,
Lit from within by raging walls of red volcanic flame,
Your terrifying face and vast sinuous body
Shine like a polished obsidian sky.

O wild joy,
Your hair and eyebrows are burning fire.
O Origin of time, of splendor, of luminous void
You have three eyes, filled with boiling blood.
Primordial luminous omniscience,
From your every glance
Shoot world-consuming lightning bolts of rage.

O all-devouring great bliss, all-devouring terror
Your steel fangs gnash with the sound of thunder.
Saliva and blood glisten on your smiling lips.
Exhausting all wisdom,
You wear a crown of five dried skulls.

O Burning Origin, O Blazing End of Life,
The wish-fulfilling jewel glows in your hair.
Origin and end of action and destruction,
You have four arms,
And with your every movement
Worlds rise, flourish, burn, and are dispersed,
As your gestures tear through the luminous heart of space.

Before anything was born,
After all has died,
Here:
You are the zero point.

As rivers of supplicants and devotees enter and leave, the visitors stand uncertainly outside. They hear the bleating of sacrificial goats, the whoosh as the knife flashes down through the air, then a tearing sound and animal gasp, and the thunk as the goat's head falls onto the ground.

They hear an old woman sing:

"Who are you?
Why is everything you do so misleading?"

——FOUR DIVINE MESSENGERS:

4 — PATH

It is said that finally Prince Siddhartha could not divert his mind from the imminence of old age, sickness, and death. There was no one to alleviate his distress. Claustrophobia engulfed him. Again he left the palace, but this time he went alone and on foot.

As sunset fell, travelers disappeared from the roads. Merchants closed their shops. Farmers withdrew into their dwellings. The air grew cool. Birds sang their lullabies before hiding in the trees. And in the deepening night, the world and its great variety of life dissolved in darkness. Prince Siddhartha wandered through the shadows of farms and forests. Animals rustled in the underbrush. Monkeys moved through the upper branches of the trees. He heard men and women sighing in their sleep, moving restlessly in dream. He heard children cry out, and old people groan. He felt time and decay and death moving like wind across the earth. The Prince sighed and suddenly felt exhausted.

The sun began to rise. He watched as, slowly, the shapes and colors of the world began to separate themselves from darkness. Birds again sang. Cattle mooed, and water buffalo roared. Men and women emerged from their dwellings and resumed their labors. "Why?" thought Prince Siddhartha, "Why this endless struggling?" He sat beside the road in the shadow of a plain tree and wept.

After some time, a beggar in tattered robes, carrying a gourd and walking with a staff, approached him. The man was young, but emaciated; his eyes were bright and alert. He looked at the Prince with detached curiosity, but said nothing. Finally, the Prince grew impatient.

"Who are you?" he asked. "Where are you going?"

"Young Lord," the beggar replied, "my name is not important since I do not seek companionship. I move from place to place, but I am not going anywhere."

The Prince was struck by the man's calm and asked: "Surely you have a family and once lived somewhere. How did you come to adopt this way of life?"

The young man took some time to answer: "As you well know, my Lord, everything alive will soon disintegrate and die. Pain does not cease. We are imprisoned here. I renounced worldly goals and set out to see what, if anything, continues."

The Prince was deeply impressed by the man's simplicity. He asked: "And, then sir, what have you found?"

"My Lord, nothing endures, but mind never ceases seeking form."

Prince Siddhartha reflected on this. He hesitated, then asked: "Is there a path beyond that?"

The beggar looked at the Prince. Time stopped. He heard the clatter of wings as a flock of blackbirds took to the air. He smelled the smoke of a wood fire. There was nothing to resist.

Then the Prince looked up. The young beggar had disappeared in the morning mist.

It was a day later when Prince Siddhartha returned to the palace. He went directly to see his father, the King. He bowed. "Great King, merciful father, please grant the request I must make. I am determined to leave the palace. For the sake of all beings, I must find the path that leads to freedom from the world of birth and death."

"Why do you think you can find something no one yet has ever found?" the King asked sadly. Prince Siddhartha could not answer. He prostrated three times to his weeping father, and left.

As he passed beneath the shadow of the great stone lintel of the palace gate, he paused. A gap opened before him. His past was behind. He had no idea where his next footstep would lead or what he would become.

Ours is a world of work unending.
That there might be some final end is not so.
Now and now, the undone must be re-done:
Inspiration must be restored
Discipline must be maintained,
The bannisters and parasols must be repaired,
Dinner, breakfast, lunch must be prepared
And eaten.
Jewels must be polished, carpets cleaned.
And gold, gold which does not change or rust,
Must be counted, hidden, stolen, shaped, and melted
    down again.
Friends must be written, condolence calls made
And love letters, true love, friendship, kind thoughts
    all nourished and renewed.

You believe, sitting as thoughts
Make you hope or squirm,
That it will stop?
That if you concentrate or relax,
Pure radiant space will sweep you clean?
You've read it, heard it, no?

But no, no, no, and no
So long as you, this world and you, endure
The work remains ever, ever undone and ever, ever, ever
To be done again.
Now.

The first time I heard Trungpa Rinpoche give a talk, I went out of curiosity. I sat in the balcony at the back of a church and waited for more than an hour. Everyone sat quietly. I didn't know if they were meditating or just waiting. Then there was whispering. People began to wander in and out of the chancel, returning to sit quietly, then stirring around, then sitting again. Eventually there was an expectant buzz. A group of nondescript young men and women bustled importantly onto the platform where Rinpoche would speak. They placed a vase of flowers and a carafe of what I later learned was rice wine on a small table to the right of a rather shabby brocade cushion, and to its left a battered armrest.

Immediately, Rinpoche limped in and sat down. He was small, stocky, and evidently crippled. His movements were slow and considered. He wore an unostentatious jacket and tie. There was nothing exotic about him. He could have been Korean or Hawaiian. But as he looked slowly at each member of the audience, his gaze was by turns indifferent, mischievous, intent, and somehow a little menacing. Seated so far back, I was relieved he could not notice me.

Rinpoche began to speak. His voice was high, a little strangled. He made no effort to flatter or charm his listeners. He scratched his neck, drank from his cup, took long pauses, smiled, drank again, resumed talking. Each gesture was uncalculated, but somehow completely conscious. I was mesmerized.

As if the space around him was fluid like water, Rinpoche's every movement unfolded and rippled in the air. When he lifted the cup, I could sense him feeling its shape, its weight; when he drank, he was aware of the temperature, the slipperiness, the taste of the sake, and when he swallowed, he followed its progress into his body. The way he put the cup down, lowering his arm slowly until the base of the cup touched the wood of the table, the small thud it made, the release of the cup's weight from his hand, made each of the gestures in this ordinary continuum magnetic. I felt I was in the presence of someone who was completely part of life.

He spoke about people not stepping into life. "You are perching on energy like a bird flitting from branch to branch."

It was a long time before I dared go see him again. In the same building, much to my shock, I bumped into him as he was leaving the men's room and I was going in. "How are you?" he asked. "Just fine," I managed. And so I began my life as his student with a lie.

In ancient times, the legendary King Indrabhuti proclaimed:

> O, you who wander in the human realm,
> On the paths of ordinary delusion,
> On the path of those who simply hear the truth,
> On the path of renunciants,
> On the path of personal realization,
> Or on any other path known thus far;
> Whether you pursue methods of purification or union,
> You struggle for liberation from bondage in samsara's
> whirling coils.

But subtly,
You conceive of enlightenment as escape;
Conceive of the infinite expanse of wakefulness
As heaven and a final resting place.

I, Indrabhuti, tell you that enlightenment is not beyond
        the world.
It is the primordial ground.
It is all-pervasive.

Unoriginated, it is the source.
Unceasing, it is extinction.
Without location, it is like space.

Because it is empty, it is the feeling of unreality.
Because it is the ground, it is the feeling of reality.
Because it is subtle, there is the experience of confusion.
Because it is unceasing, there is the experience of meaning.
Because it is non-dual, it is complete compassion.
Because it is compassion, it is the truth and the innate law.

Logic does not capture or penetrate it.
Renunciation does not purify it.
Meditation does not stabilize it.
Behavior does not expand or diminish it.
It is reality itself and is not an attainment of any kind.

Moving from realm to realm
By awareness, by vision, by living,
By caring for the well-being of all who live,
By loving them;
All this is the same as the light of the sun
Passing through clouds.

I dream I am on a journey I have long wanted to take. I am sitting at the cave's opening. I look out over a narrow valley. The pine trees look black, and I gaze at the branches of trees whose leaves have fallen lower in the ravine. Huge slabs of granite, gray and cracked, rise from the floor far below. I hear a racing creek at the bottom, but I cannot see it. A light snow with large puffy flakes, the first of the winter, emerges out of the gray air with a faint hiss, floats and falls, disappears below.

I dream I am wearing a rough wool robe and sitting on an antelope skin. I have set up a small shrine against the dry rock wall to my left. A table in front holds the two texts I will practice, my vajra, bell, and kapala. Deeper in the cave is an old trunk with sacks of grain. A small fire flutters with air moving out from somewhere deep in the earth.

In sleep, I hear the purling of the stream fading in the air from far below. Outside, the cold breeze carries a hint of incense. Perhaps I am imagining it. All who practiced here before me have left some momentum, a slender and enduring stream which now is carrying me. I feel overwhelmed. My teachers have drawn this stream into the world. It is carrying me.

I look out into the evening sky. I imagine myself hurtling through the air, the earth and sky spinning around me. Air rushing, tearing at my arms and legs, pulling my hair, ripping at my clothes. Exhilaration and terror. The swirling, looming earth, and the inescapable violent pain, unimaginable. Some transformation, end and intensity beyond any mind.

§ § §

Since the instant of your birth
You are being transformed.
It is your path.
It is making you.

There is the solitude of one self.
One self is sitting in a room in shadow.
There is the life that is pulsing from within and pushing
Pushing out
Out into uncertain night
Where a loving consort waits
Where there may be an assassin
Where the crickets are singing under the floor
Where a child is dying alone
Where a farmer is turning home exhausted
Where there is no rice
Where there is a wonderful book
Where another man nearby has a great deal of rice
Where a woman is giving birth
Where a fox is biting the hen's neck
Where the god of thunder wakes
Where the goddess in an apple tree spreads her legs
Where a frog dives into the depths of a pond
Where an old man drinks rice wine and waits,
Wondering if waiting to write corrupts the night,
Returning to sit in the shadows.

There is the chaos of meditation
Where there is the discomfort of solitude
The waiting for a guest who does not arrive
The visitor who one hears outside on the path,
Who refuses to answer.

Long ago, the great Indian teacher, Kanha, sang this song of the path:

When moving through reality, like space,
The desire to go anywhere
Is a ghost's quest to reach the horizon.
Wishing to get to the juicy conclusion
You're a deer chasing the water-mirage.

You've been Buddha from the beginning!
Big mistake to become Buddha again.

Why would you think
You can recreate the enlightenment of someone else?

In one of Trungpa Rinpoche's early seminars, he talked about goal and path in this way:

"The goal exists in every moment of our life situation on our spiritual journey. In this way, the spiritual journey becomes equally exciting and beautiful. As if you are Buddha already. There are constant new discoveries, constant messages, and constant warnings. Constantly cutting down. Constant painful as well as pleasurable lessons... It is a complete journey... It doesn't have to be labeled 'spirituality' as such."

When Prince Siddhartha had stood before his father, and King Suddhodana had tried to dissuade him from departing, the Prince could find no way to explain. He could not capture the torrent of words and images that were passing through him. Time alone would make these appear. From teacher to student, from mouth to ear, the wordless would become an unending stream of moments, a boundless sea of true love's clarity, opening like a luminous white lotus, a lineage endlessly unfolding from the depths of space.

THE EMPTY ROOM

For Tatiana Alekseevna Mikhailova

I

I dreamed I wandered through a dense, light-dappled rainforest. At a bend in the path, I found myself suddenly on the banks of a sluggish stream. Across the stream, in deeper shadows, I saw a twig hut with a palm-leaf roof. An old woman, cross-eyed, with dark, dusty skin, and dirty, matted hair, sat on the ground in front of the hut. Her half-demented smile as she glanced up at me revealed a mouth full of broken teeth. With a skeletal right hand, she lifted a copper water pot to her mouth and drank. The water dribbled from the corners of her mouth, down her neck, and along her dried-up breasts.

She hummed contentedly to herself. Suddenly she looked directly at me. She stared and leered as she ran her black tongue slowly across her cracked lips.

I was embarrassed. I felt like a peeping-tom, and was filled with indecision, even panic. I did not want to be involved in any way with this crazy person, but I was caught by a certain disgusted fascination. My only alternative was to run away, but that would be even more embarrassing.

As I stood there fixed, all at once I noticed an enormous tiger prowling fluidly through the shadows, moving slowly towards the woman from behind her hut. I had seen tigers before, locked in cages, chained at palace gates, and even in the wild from far off. But nothing prepared me for the immense sinuous power of the beast, or the splendid opulence of its black stripes and orange fur. I felt myself reflected in the predatory intelligence of its golden eyes. I thought I could feel the heat of its blood-scented breath, pulsing past the gleaming fangs and hard black lips, burning on my face.

Unconcerned as the tiger crept close behind her, the old woman continued to stare at me, running her left hand up and down the inside of her thigh in a revolting and unmistakable gesture of sexual invitation.

Before I could react or shout a warning, the tiger shot out from the underbrush and leapt into the air. In one bound, the beast flew over the old woman, over the flat earth where she sat, over the river, and dropped, hot mouth gaping, engulfing me. I passed out and felt I was swallowed into the black steaming void of the creature's maw. I was tumbling in the dark, beyond fear, pain, death. The tiger had devoured me, the old woman, the hut, the jungle, everything.

I felt a stream of cool water trickle down my throat, and I woke. My head lay in the hag's lap. Seen up close, her dark skin glowed like polished leather. She smelled pleasantly of cinnamon. She smiled tenderly at me as she carefully poured water from the copper pot onto my lips. The tiger, calm and majestic, sat curled around the hag at her back. From time to time, he idly licked her shoulder, leaving a slight trail of spit. Though everything was simple and clear, I was confused.

"There isn't any mystery here," said the hag in a soft, light, youthful voice. "You experienced this."

II

The stream of the dreaming mind breaks through into the light of early morning. She cannot use her bathroom. There is a woman in there. She knows this. She waits for a long time. Finally, she makes her way down the crooked stairs to the basement. "I made a little bathroom down there," she explains to her daughter. The daughter looks in the bathroom. The light is on, but there is no one there. The toilet has not been flushed.

There's no one there, Mother.
There was a woman... I thought there was... What was I thinking?
Where's Daddy?
He's dead, Mom.
Really?
He's been dead for 20 years.
I guess I knew that.
You did. You do.
They're all dead, aren't they?
                    Why is it everyone I ask about is dead?

Dream and wake — all that she loved in the living, all that was familiar, all that made up the problems to be solved, the uncertainty, the regularity of things, the secret desires, the secret regrets, the questions, all these have moved to the realm of the dead, and emerge into waking life now on the rivulets of dream. They flow out into the day; under the hard light of day they soften, making a reality like quicksand. Daily life and the night world of the dead are merging, so much easier now to lose her way, easier now to sink into things that before were simply flickering thoughts. Now returned as shadow in light, as permeability, directionless.

Is she the nameless woman in the bathroom, or is it her sister, so long gone but so vivid, so part of a life continuing. The living, the dead.

She moves in the borderland where there is no path. You must remember, they say. Why?

She moves in the... not swamp... what is the word... the marshes, lost amid their tall reeds. And walking, she suddenly surprises a huge blue heron which clatters in flight up, up in ungainly flight.

No, that's a memory. She was walking with her father. She was little, small.

Now still small.

Who was that small woman who was just here? She asks her daughter.
Who do you mean?
The small woman.
You're a small woman.
No, it's not me.

Real, not real.
She can't explain it.
She is curious.
Why is she thinking these things?
They are taking her away, the way they took the car.

§ § §

Even as the world is fading, our bodies are losing color, our features are losing their distinction.

Even as the impulse forward weakens, we do not find rest, cannot rest in the shapes the present is offering, past and homeland now unanchored, floating.

It is a time of estrangement.

We are no longer the wanderer in the landscape so much as the mist in a landscape of undiminished vividness.

This mist is not obscuration, but an elusive moment, a transient focus, ambient pain, sorrow, thoughts that have clustered but cannot quite coalesce.

We no longer have the illusion that we will shape the
world, own it, cleave to it, articulate it.
The flow will not be directed, banked up, dammed.
Its momentary uniqueness can no longer be expressed,
shared, given
By one to another,
From one moment to the next.
To remain within the conventions of core and extension
takes far more effort.
One's mind-traffic is no longer so easily subject to the
arbitrary traffic lights, the painted lines, the
arrows, STOP and NO and YES.

I don't care, said my mother-in-law who always cared
Couldn't care less, said the teacher who always cared
I don't give a fuck, said my father who never swore
We were hurrying through a crowded airport

It feels so often that a story is about to begin. We are waiting.

A memory, almost from a different life, clear and vivid like the smell of gasoline, appears, disappears.

An outcast bar-girl,
A secret yogini,
The Dombhi
Is imprisoned.
And bliss pervades her form.
Inner channels shine:
No word can enter in.

There is no disentangling
What fools call sense,
What fools call non-sense.

A woman alone on a tired sofa in the fading light: medicines, poisons in their own right, pour through her veins. Not comfortable, not exactly painful, but continuously exhausting. She is being cured and depleted simultaneously. Her taste is gone, supplanted by a flat ugly scent, like smoke above a battlefield. She is not actually thinking, but all kinds of thoughts move through her. She does not react, but sometimes, for no apparent reason, finds herself sobbing.

Long, long ago, the yogi Kanhapada sang:

My body is compassion,
The inner room is vacant.

I crossed the world-sea in a dream of illusion.
Wave piled on wave,
And I was adrift.
There was no shore and no escape.

Awareness rows on.

Now,
Across the sea of successive illusions,
Smell, touch, seeing, hearing, taste
Do not change
Like dreams without sleep.

We knocked on the door of an old friend who had recently recovered from a stroke.

There had been some confusion in the emails about when we would arrive. We waited a long time before she opened the door. She showed us in. Clearly things were not going as well as they might. Things weren't as tidy as they once were. She looked at me sharply.

"You know, I never expected to see you alive again."

I smiled, and felt I might have stepped into a slightly altered realm. I was about to say: "Maybe you were right," but thought better of it.

§ § §

We often visit Munich where my wife, Deborah, lived for 22 years, teaching clarinet at the Richard Strauss Conservatory and the Hochschule für Musik, and played in the Bayerische Rundfunk Symphonieorchester. Visits to Munich are like going home and seeing her large musical family in this elegant, artistic, prosperous, and most civilized city. On our last visit, for no reason I can discern, people spoke openly about their experiences during WWII.

They were not from the generation that remembered much of politics; their earliest memories concerned surviving bombings and living in ruins. Such memories surfaced unexpectedly to innocent prompts. "What a beautiful piece of furniture," I stood in front of an old marquetry cabinet. "Oh," said our hostess, "It was the only thing that was left after my grandfather's house was bombed." I must have looked a little shocked. "Well, you and your family, you too must have suffered at that time," she said. "No. No, we didn't," was all I could reply.

Her husband showed me a painting, a sort of mediocre pallid Cézanne-derived picture of some scrubby shrubs next to a wall. I recognized it as the sort of paintings he'd shown me that his father had made: they all had a kind of determined uneventfulness. "It's your father's," I said. "Yes. He painted it while he was in the army occupying Paris, and on the same day he first met my mother." I was staggered. Here, hidden deep in this nondescript object, were concealed moments of great intensity. Munich itself, rebuilt extensively after being bombed, is somewhat like this. Here and there a whiff of sulfur still remains. The building where my wife taught was once the Führerbau. Here I began to feel that in the continuity of things hides secrets that only come to life on the edge of sleep. So, you, even if all we know were to be changed beyond recognition, something would still emerge.

——DIE GLEISE (THE TRACKS)
BENEATH A CITY AFTER WAR

For Deborah Marshall

Beneath the city at varying depths: seams of granite, subterranean water courses, cables, rusting pipes, underground trains, linkages spread under the surface of the earth carrying water, energy, waste, men, women, ambitions, daydreams, plans, terrors, memories, fatigue. Such are the neurons linking the impulses of a city, binding the city's ever-changing surface to the density of its dark geology.

A middle-aged man in a soiled raincoat sits on a bench in the underground train. He is lost in thought, rocked by rhythmic crashing as the train hurtles through the dark. He looks down and turns the pages of a book by Athanasius Kircher that he had just found in a used bookstore. He bought the book because of this quote: "This world is bound with secret knots." Now he cannot find the citation. He looks up.

Across from him, a woman is looking at a pamphlet of an art exhibit in Vienna. On the cover is the detail of a watercolor showing dense columns of dark blue water descending on a pale landscape. Everyone on the train is sitting silently. Some read, some consult their phones, some simply look forward.

GLEIS 1

The pamphlet of the exhibit bears the following quote:

"At night, in early summer, I was asleep yet saw clearly as many great floods cascaded from the sky. The first flood struck the earth about four miles away with terrible force. A great roar and crashing, as the whole land was drowned, and all farms washed away, and all human habitations ripped up. And there were many other floods further away, but all coming from the sky like huge seas. They came down from a great height, but all seemed to fall slowly, slowly. Then, after the first wave struck and began to approach, water fell with such swiftness, wind and roaring, that I woke trembling. I had seen the end of the world. For a long while I could not come to my senses. When I arose in the morning I painted what I had seen. May God turn all things to the best."

–Albrecht Dürer, 1525

GLEIS 2

At the beginning of spring, the Plague began to show itself. It began in both men and women with certain swellings both in the groin and the armpits, some of which grew to the size of a normal apple or the size of an egg. Within a brief space of time, these deadly swellings began to spread indiscriminately over every part of the body. After this, the symptoms changed to black or livid spots, sometimes large, sometimes small, all over the body. The swellings, as well as the spots, were signs of impending death.

Few survived the illness, and most died three days after the appearance of the above symptoms without any fever or other side effects. The power of this plague was so great that it passed by contact not only from one person to another, but also by contact with the possessions of an afflicted person. I myself saw the clothes of one who died from the Plague cast on the street where two pigs took them in their mouths, and by the afternoon they died as if the rags had been poisoned. From occurrences such as these, all who were well came to take a very cruel attitude towards those who were ill, shunning them, sealing them in their houses, and avoiding them by all possible means.

All the laws, whether of gods or man, fell into disuse. The living, the dead, the yet unborn mingled. Sometimes they saw each other, sometimes not. Definitions, borders, limits became unknown. As in a dream, all merged, transformed, disappeared like shapes seen in offering smoke.

GLEIS 3

Centuries later, fortunes restored, the Prince, who ruled the city and its surroundings, was a prodigal collector of art, and he heard of Dürer's large vellum notebook in which the artist's dream and painting were recorded. His agents were unable to obtain it, but made a copy of this world-ending division.

At the same time, however, his agents found a singular object he had heard of long before, and since then desired: a crystal the height of a man's index finger with a circumference twice that of a man's thumb. It is completely clear with a slightly grayish cast, and only a few bubbles. But within, there is a horned devil, black and tiny, with arms, legs, and a tail frozen in rage. It is said that a renowned exorcist captured this demon when he drew it from a woman who had killed her child.

The train stops. A thin, gray-haired woman in a long maroon wool coat bustles on, pushing a baby carriage in which a tiny child sleeps. She takes a seat and begins to read to herself from a book of children's stories.

GLEIS 4

It was a golden autumn afternoon. A magistrate in a small mountain town was in his study reviewing some records when a servant reported that a man dressed in black had just entered the courtyard. The man was wearing a black silk pillbox hat, and led a sleek black horse. On the horse's back was an object shaped like a cushion, covered in black horse hide. The man in black took the object off the horse's back and set it on the ground.

The black pillow then began rolling across the courtyard, casting a long shadow as it moved. It rolled up the steps, entered the magistrate's study, and bounced up on his knees.

The magistrate wanted to run but could not move. He looked in horror as the skin covering the pillow then peeled back on all sides like a huge black rose unfolding. Inside, the object was completely lined with eyes. They were alive. They blinked, rolled, and winked as they looked around in all directions. The magistrate was frozen, terrified, but he could not look away. The eyes kept looking in all directions.

After a long time, the pillow closed. It rolled off the magistrate's knees and went back out to the courtyard. The man in black replaced it on the horse. The magistrate woke, as from a dream, and he ordered the servant to follow, but the man in black, the horse, and the strange object all had vanished.

The magistrate could not shake the dread which had consumed him. He entered a monastery, but to no avail.

Another stop. Tourists, three women, and a man enter, sit, and unfold a map. The man, thin, long blondish hair, wearing a blue down jacket, gets up to consult the subway map next to the door. He returns to his companions, and they reach a tentative agreement. A young woman turns away from her companions and reads from a guidebook.

GLEIS 5

Farmers have lived for centuries in the lush emerald valleys, high in the mountains surrounding the city. They raise wheat, pigs, cattle, sheep; they make bread, ham, cheese, wool.

The mountains that tower around them glow with celestial brilliance amid white translucent clouds in the blazing summer sun. They shine like rock crystals. Blinding light reflects off the sheer rock planes, white and pure as air. White light radiates without direction, binds the mountains and the sky.

The farmers are proud and cautious about the power of these mountains and their light.

But this immense luminosity, this unimpeded vastness, can take possession of a visitor. A frustrated artist found his mind and his ambitions soaring, sparked to a scale previously unimaginable. This light, this rising upward, seeing it, joining it. It has an inhuman power. Speaking of it has power. The failed art student rose to notoriety as a man of politics, a rabble-rouser inspiring those who live in the city's darkness. Violence, warfare, slaughter, destruction, all can be encompassed in this light. Intoxicated with light, he led men past all constraint or law.

Cruelty, murder, war, death and torture all followed. Intoxicated, or afraid, they followed.

GLEIS 6

A strange painting for a Prince to covet, but when he heard of it, he was willing to pay anything, despite his councilors' anxious warnings that the treasury could no longer withstand such extravagances. He always kept it nearby.

The catalogue of the forced sale of his possessions still exists. In it, the painting is described this way: Oil on canvas.

Quite large. A scene in late autumn. The sky is gray, the land exhausted. A weary farmer in a torn canvas smock leads a starving horse. It pulls a broken wooden wagon full of dry hay. They are passing by some goats who wander in the remains of a great hall, its walls fallen in, its roof collapsed. Ahead of them is a burned and barren orchard, the trunks of trees scorched black and lifeless. In the background, an old woman sits, her back against the ruins of a church, its apse broken in like an eggshell.

GLEIS 7

In the last year of his life, the prodigal Prince paid a small fortune for a little painting, perhaps 300 years old. The oil on wood still had the hard, bright surface of an enamel. The entirety of the square panel is covered with irregular layers of green trees and shadows, a horizonless and impenetrable forest rendered in minute detail.

Dwarfed in the lower right-hand corner, the tiny figure of Saint George battles a dragon.

The Prince sighed: "We want to forget that anyone who ventured beyond his village was soon lost in a deep forest. Lost, alone, how many travelers found themselves in mortal struggles with demons that those who stay home do not imagine."

A young woman, dark-haired and flushed, writes intently on a piece of cream-colored note paper: "I want to tell you how much I love you. How near it feels, my conclusion, an unraveling, which leaves skeins of color and sound, disembodied tree smells, body smells, floating out with no vector or return. Going, this word I, going. And you whom I love. I am a breeze touching you, unanchored continuing love. It is not holding together, but extending."

GLEIS 8

Generations later, the principality's fortunes revived, the current Prince decided to build a cathedral that would be the greatest in Christendom. He asked builders to submit plans and estimates of costs. All understood that should the winning builder fail to fulfill his promises, he would be executed and his family exiled. Nonetheless, many were still confident enough to make proposals. The Prince chose the builder who promised a structure that was the largest, most beautiful, and, decisively, the least costly.

It was early winter. The construction of the cathedral was well under way when the builder realized he would run out of funds long before the project was complete. He was in despair and did not know what to do.

The Devil always slides through a hairline of uncertainty, and he now appeared before the anxious builder as a kindly old priest. He promised limitless funds if, for his part, the builder promised to complete the cathedral without windows. He wanted the cathedral, as he said, to be "eyeless." Should he fail, the devil would take the builder's soul to dwell in blinding torment for all eternity.

The builder had no choice but to agree. What else could he do? And suddenly, like a lightning bolt from an empty sky, the Pope in Rome made a huge contribution to complete the cathedral, and promised more if needed. The builder hired more laborers and purchased more costly materials for the church's interior. Construction now moved along quickly. The builder now devoted himself to devising a way to escape the consequences of his pledges. And, because virtue has no less guile than sin, his calculations soon showed him the way.

One fragrant night in early spring, just before the cathedral's grand opening when the Prince, the Papal Nuncio, great nobles from far and wide, constables, professors, and all the powerful merchants were to arrive, the Devil made an early inspection. Now he appeared as he really is, long and wiry, black as night, with eyes of burning coals, teeth of steel tines, his long razor-sharp tail flicking impatiently, and a stench of burning sulfur swirling about him. His voice was silky and beautiful.

"So?... Show me." The builder managed not to tremble as he showed the Devil where to stand. It was the one place in the vast building where, due to the placement of columns and the altar screen, no windows were visible. "Good...Very good."

"You agree, I have fulfilled my side of the bargain?"

"True. You have." But just then the sun began to rise. Faint light began to leak into the cathedral.

"But what is this?" the Devil hissed.

"It's only a little light. As you know more than most, nothing in this world is perfect." But now sunlight was pouring into the church, even if the Demon could not see how. The Devil screamed and seethed. His body became hot as a burning iron, and with a terrible stench his footprint burned deep into the marble floor. The Devil moved from the one spot that hid the windows. He saw how he had been deceived.

"You dare to cheat me! Do you not know who I am?" The Devil flew into the air in a shower of sparks.

"But, Great Evil One though you may be, still you are bound by the word you've given." And the builder was about to say more, but quickly thought better of it. The Devil burst into flame and dissolved in a cloud of smoke.

The consecration of the cathedral soon began with dazzling pomp and splendor greater than anyone had ever seen. The Prince was more pleased than he had imagined, and granted the builder the title of Master Builder to the Prince with an income in perpetuity.

The builder accepted the money, but politely declined the honors. Next year he moved his family to a distant country.

The Devil's black footprint with its tiny trail of flame remained burned into the cathedral's marble floor at the very spot where he had stood and been deceived.

An older woman, composed, well dressed in a gray wool suit, looks straight forward, oblivious to the others in the train, the noise. The fluorescent lights flicker briefly, and she looks up. Very near here, above ground, in a cold autumn afternoon long ago, a little girl in a nightdress and an overcoat used a spoon to dig a hole behind a bank of dormant rose bushes near the stone garden wall. The rose thorns tore her skirt. Water seeped through her felt slippers. She buried a little box that held the ring and a bracelet that her grandmother had given her.

GLEIS 9

It was the middle of a dazzling hot summer. All waited amid reports and rumors about coming armies, and worse, plagues now suddenly erupting. All awaited the approach of death and sickness that might be crossing mountains, moving through air, festering in garbage, in outhouses, cisterns. Some emblem of fate concealed deep within the whorls on a fingerprint, the spit of a traveler, the excrement of a refugee, the hair of a woman. They were waiting for unimaginable transformations to engulf them. They gathered in the dark church to pray. They sang:

Death is at hand.
Our senses fail.
Our tongues are dumb;
Now, O God, prevail.

Lo! Satan strains
To snatch his prey;
We feel his grasp;
Must we now our souls betray?

O God, let sin no more.
Keep us in the bonds of strife;
Lift us up, You whom we adore
Straight into the skies of life.

GLEIS 10

Many still remember that early autumn. The sky above the center of the city was without color and without clouds. The war was nearing its end. No defenses were left. The air, suddenly, was completely silent. Everyone looked up. A flock of huge blackbirds circled slowly; suddenly they vanished into the empty sky.

Bombs rained down, whistling and shrieking, exploding, bursting into flame. The city and all its splendid buildings, its fountains, squares, marketplaces, all were shattered. Some walls remained standing, but in the choking clouds of powder and dust, nothing remained familiar.

The cathedral's roof had collapsed, all its windows no longer existed. The Devil's footprint remained and seemed now slightly larger.

The brakes squeal as the train turns. The old woman shakes her head. The man in the soiled raincoat, flipping through the pages of an old book, stops and reads the cryptic sentence: "It does not change in time." He pauses to think. A teenaged boy, blond, wearing ragged jeans and an expensive green leather jacket, looks at his cell phone, then stares through the window at his reflection hovering in the dark tunnel.

The train stops, and a half-dozen African women, two quite thin but most of them ample, burst laughing onto the train. The other passengers stare openly. They are dressed for a wedding celebration. They wear floor-length gowns of lace over dazzling brocades of scarlet, lilac, saffron, emerald. They are carrying gifts in golden wrapping paper, and cakes in white boxes. They are going to church in what was once a police station. They gossip and giggle. They smell like tropical flowers. The train rocks gently as it hurtles through the dark. They have come from a distant and terrifying land. They know they will not feel at home here. It is all alien. They are giddy to find themselves so unafraid.

§ § §

*O*n the night of the 2016 election, I happened to have dinner with my friend Emilio. We hadn't seen each other for a long time, and he invited me to La Grenouille. It was the last restaurant in New York to serve French haute cuisine of the kind popular in the 1970s, and had a kind of secure opulence no longer common.

There were protestors marching on Fifth Avenue a few yards away, but within all was peaceful with the clink of silverware, the buzz of contentment, the scent of cut flowers, women's perfume, beurre blanc. Flushed faces shone in the pink table lamps. Our waiter moved smoothly, but was perhaps a little tense. He chatted about the wine with Emilio in Spanish. He was, it turned out, Mexican.

"And what do you think the customers are thinking about?" I asked Emilio.

"The seas and seas of money they'll soon be swimming in," he said.

I told him I was thinking of writing about the subliminal influence of impending ecological collapse. He nodded. Four well-dressed customers came into the restaurant laughing; suddenly the aggrieved shouts of the nearby marchers were not muffled. Emilo said: "It's happening again."

PATHS IN GATHERING DARKNESS

It becomes clear, as we move into old age, that the world is moving away from us. It is no longer possible for us to leap into the world, as children do, and try to seize it. It is no longer for us to work at forming ourselves, to find how to join the world, to embrace it. This we did as young women and men. The time when we strive to shape the world, to hold it in our grasp, to pass it on, all this is no longer possible. This cannot be helped. We feel it all moving away, and with that comes a great gift of seeing new landscapes, new patterns, feeling new intensities, new love, new gratitude. There is an expanded display, a deeper response to colors and smells and tastes, and a tenderness we could not have imagined. The world seems to expand as we feel ourselves contract.

The world others create around us means less and less. As younger people, we aimed to find and make our place in the adult world in which we were growing up. That world now is unknown to younger people, its values not dismissed, but no longer recognized. Our accomplishments, our sensibility, are part of a domain that has vanished. Our teachers, the friends with whom we shared our journey, all are gone. And there is no anchor even for nostalgia. What we have cared for fades away in the roar of the all-encompassing present.

Now our senses begin to fail. We cannot hear; ambient space loses its dimensions. We are not sure of understanding what is said. We talk so that we don't have to pretend to hear. Our seeing fades, our senses of taste and smell flatten. The civilized control of bodily functions that has allowed us to be adults falters. We become "management issues" for others. Our memories, even if they were now relevant, begin to dissolve. Who are we now? And what?

What did my mother say when she arrived in the emergency room having drunk too much, fallen, hit her head, and been picked up by the ambulance?

"I demand an autopsy."

In 1979, just before the Lunar New Year, Chögyam Trungpa Rinpoche wrote a private letter to two students who asked to be sent to another teacher. The two, husband and wife, felt they had reached an impasse in their study and practice. Their path seemed suddenly to have hit a wall. Rinpoche, as he said, was shocked at how they felt. He wrote:

> "I hope you will understand I have a certain integrity and sense of belief. My existence is not just based on the logic of growing up, becoming educated, getting married, having a job, bringing up children, and then dropping dead. ... As you well understand, even if I were tortured to death, I would never give up my cause, my respect for my teacher, and my heritage... what I say and feel is true, there is nothing hidden."

Nonetheless, he was puzzled.

Even now, almost 40 years later, these words seem nakedly simple and painfully blunt. Even if one is inclined to find the "even if I were tortured to death" overly dramatic, one might reflect that this was indeed the recent fate of Trungpa Rinpoche's own teachers. What strikes us now as almost embarrassing is the openness with which Rinpoche could state his life's purpose and meaning. And throughout his life he placed great emphasis on the earliest teachings of the Buddha. He returned again and again to the Buddha's search for the truth that lies within the constant confusions and emotional upheavals of daily life, and he often referred to the Buddha's earliest formulations of his discovery. Throughout Trungpa Rinpoche's life of exile and wandering, these teachings remained the lodestar.

The Buddha spent years of his life examining the nature of existence. He explored the innate qualities and dispositions of mind, of being, of the universe. He did not learn from a book or a god or a super-human entity. He proceeded by direct and exhaustive examination of his own experience. Pervading all phenomena, within all aspects of mind, like water flowing through a dense forest, he discovered the unceasing light of the awakened state. His former fellow seekers asked him to explain, and it took him seven weeks to formulate a way to guide them. What he taught them was how to live in the world where change and the unchanging, delusion and clarity, selfishness and compassion, bondage and liberation, are intertwined.

As the great 13th century-master Dogen Zenji put it: "...if you search for a buddha outside birth and death... you will cause yourself to remain all the more in birth and death, and lose the way to liberation... birth and death is the life of a Buddha."

The Buddha's teachings are not a method for transforming a less desirable state of mind into a more desirable one. They are, purely and simply, a way of continually exploring what is. The essence of what the Buddha discovered, and the core of what he then taught, are the Four Noble Truths. These are called truths because they are not the result of inference. They are true on their own merits and as a matter of circumstance. They are the discoveries of direct observation. When we look at life, without adding or subtracting anything, these are what we see. What is special here, and hence "Noble," is that the Buddha found the great value in what we usually do not wish to acknowledge. He presented these truths as doorways and paths in the world of our imprisonment and, simultaneously, our liberation. Everything in our lives, from birth to death and beyond, is worthy to be an element of our path.

The First Noble Truth is that the nature of existence is suffering, pain, anxiety, and dissatisfaction. We cannot prevent continuous discomfort, sickness, old age, death. We want to have security, pleasure, esteem. The feeling of wanting is painful. And when we get what we desire, we change or whatever we sought changes. The truth of the matter is that we cannot maintain, hold on to, or make permanent anything in our lives. And we cannot escape the anxiety caused by fear, loss, pain, and death.

We, the aging and the old, are entering an alien land. It is as if we are now moving into a delta where a river joins the sea. There are thousands of tiny islands. We find ourselves engulfed in ever denser mists and fog, moving uncertainly from isle to isle. There is no solid ground nor landscape that does not shift and change.

The Second Noble Truth, the origin of this suffering, is that we are always trying to make and remake ourselves and our world. We are always searching for pleasure, satisfaction, and stable ways of being. We are constantly trying to find forms of thought and belief in which we can find refuge. Seeking control over ourselves and our circumstances, we feel anguish that we cannot find them. The first truth refers to impermanence and dissolution, while the second concerns illusion and birth. The two move together. They weave and unweave in the fabric of the mind and senses.

The world arounds us dissolves, reforms, now in more pallid tones. And in the same way we feel we are dissolving and reforming. Reaching and reforming. We struggle to continue what less and less we understand.

The Third Noble Truth is cessation. Here is the ever-present continuum of deep awareness that never changes, even amid change. Amid sound it is silence. Amid ever shifting clouds it is the sky. It is beyond all concepts and conventions. It is awareness not constrained by words or thought processes or sensation. In the earliest of the Buddha's discourses, the Buddha describes this as "the unborn, un-aging, un-ailing, deathless, sorrowless, undefiled supreme security from bondage." It is "profound, hard to see, hard to understand… unattainable by mere reasoning."

The Fourth Noble Truth is called the Eight-Fold Path. It provides a detailed and concrete way of discovering the preceding truths anew. The Eight-Fold Path is not a code of inner and outer behaviors we impose on our lives to make things orderly, predictable, and less painful. It is not a set of concepts we can apply to our confusion and sorrow in order to achieve an ideal or goal. The teachings in the Eight-Fold Path are like eight stepping-stones hidden just below the moving surface of a racing stream. The Buddha discovered this path by looking directly at his mind and world, by peeling away layer after layer of emotional biases and conventional concepts. The Buddha did not look away from terror, uncertainty, longing, abandonment, despair. He did cling to conclusions. He looked into his hopes, fears, fantasies, and all else. He waited without hope of succeeding, and his attention did not waver.

At heart, to follow the Buddha's path is not just to follow the Buddha's words. Following the Buddha's path, we continue his searching in circumstances that are always new to us. And we do not know exactly who we change, and life changes around us. The Buddha's discoveries are only meaningful when discovered as new, alive.

The Eight-Fold Path emerges from what is innate in our experience. Clarity, Yearning for clarity, Awareness of convention's deceit, Free to put intention into practice, Not limited by the need to survive, Able to search, Able to discern what is real, Able to let be what unfolds beyond knowing, beyond hope and fear. We've all touched on such moments at one time or another. Right View, Right Intention, Right Speech, Right Action, Right Livelihood, Right Effort, Right Mindfulness, and Right Meditation are the outgrowth and embodiment of these moments. They are, as has been shown by the Buddha and his successors, the stepping-stones though all confusion and darkness.

Aging, being sick without a possible recovery, and dying, we are entering a new terrain. We do not know what it is. We do not know what we are experiencing. So, as we move through the dark night of life's end, chaos of bodily collapse and mental instability, another reality pulses, opens, closes. It has us in its grip. We try to wriggle out of it. As we enter the twisting paths of the dark forest, we cannot know what, if any, is the best way to proceed, or if any kind of control is available to us. We cannot say if we will stay on a path or lose our way; and if we lose our way, we cannot know if we will realize that we are lost. At this point, such chaos, such devastation, such uncertainty is our only ground.

The legendary 10th-century Buddhist yogi Tilopa, a sesame seed grinder and brothel attendant, was often found sitting on a riverbank, naked and filthy, eating raw fish. To address such depths of confusion, he summarized the path in six words, which translated are:

Don't live in the past
Don't imagine the future
Don't think of the present
Don't analyze
You can't control anything
Let go

Following these teachings, when our lives, at the end, are coming apart, as our minds are spinning into utter chaos, are we not simply diving into what is already happening? We are not trying to escape. We cannot. Is this then not an expression of supreme confidence in the nature of existence altogether? Is this not accepting the compassion of what has given us birth, sustained us, and now consumes us utterly? Nouns, verbs, sentences no longer provide guard-rails. We have never been, and are not now, nor ever will be, separate from vast, unending fields of light. Or nothing completely.

Nor is this situation in any way different from what we encounter at the time of our birth.

§ § §

The day after the 2016 election, I had lunch with Emma and James who were the presiding forces at Tricycle. They are both sensitive and thoughtful. We met in a small lunch restaurant; the atmosphere was subdued.

"I want to write about the widespread apprehension that the world might end."

"That's reasonable," James laughed. (This thought developed into a 2017 essay for Tricycle entitled A World Ever At Its End.)

*"But how do you and people of your generation think
of this sense of impending catastrophe?" I asked Emma, who
was in her late 20s.*

*She took her time but didn't hesitate: "Despair, and an
absence of any kind of model."*

*From this reply emerged several essays, including the
preceding one and that which follows. The notion of "model"
was the inspiration for the essays about two exemplary heroes.
Both lost their lives, and neither created situations that prevailed,
nonetheless they upheld their commitments to the teachings and
their followers.*

*After I left our luncheon, I wandered into the bookstore
at the nearby Rubin Museum. Lots of bright orientalia. I opened
a book and read:*

*"The elements do not have the essential nature
That you think they possess;
Since you are so deeply ignorant of this world,
How could you correctly realize anything about the world beyond?"*

THE EMPTY BOAT

I

Once upon a time, a group of men and women wished to find the one thing that would fulfill every desire. They had heard of the mythical wish-fulfilling jewel, a huge diamond that radiated dazzling light and granted absolute freedom from impoverishment, suffering, doubt, and fear to those who possess it. They became obsessed with it. They knew from ancient texts that they would have to traverse thousands of miles of treacherous and desolate mountain trails, but the prospect of such hardship, terror, and sickness only strengthened their resolve. The treasure they sought would more than make up for even the worst kinds of suffering. A life devoid of uncertainty, a life marked only by luxury and ease, was more than worth a limited period of intense hardship. Soon after they had decided they would devote their lives to this quest, the group was fortunate that a guide, a man renowned for his honesty and intelligence, who had explored and dwelt in many of the most remote regions of the world, was visiting nearby. They arranged a meeting, and were delighted to find that the guide was planning to visit the snow-capped mountains very close to the group's intended goal. He agreed to lead them, and after a few weeks' preparation they all set forth.

The trails that were easy at first became ever more steep, more treacherous, more bleak. Mild weather turned cold, freezing, windy. Howls of wolves and the roaring of bears filled the nights. Vultures tracked their progress by day. Weeks became months, and months became years, and the seekers were often hungry and always exhausted. Some sickened and died, others fell by the path and did not go on. No matter what, the guide moved steadily ahead, never saying a word. The seekers followed and kept up their spirits by speculating on their future happiness and finding ways to dismiss their doubts; the more educated took delight in petty philosophical disputes. All of them yearned for sleep, food, sex, wealth, and fame. Even so, they became disheartened. They came to doubt that any treasure could be worth such suffering.

They said to their guide: "This is futile. We cannot go on. The goal is so far off. We want to turn back."

None of this surprised the guide. He had experience with many groups of seekers. He knew people's minds as well as he knew the harsh terrain through which they had to pass. A deep well of love and affection for those who had so trusted him rose up in him; he didn't want them to have suffered so much in vain. And, he was a man of many skillful stratagems, determined that they should attain their goal. He said: "Don't be afraid! Soon we will reach a city where you can stop and rest. Later, when you have the strength, we can continue. Surely, then you will find the treasure you seek." Thus encouraged, the group continued.

The very next day they saw a splendid and powerful city with high crimson walls and bronze gates at the far end of a peaceful valley. Just the sight of it revived the weary travelers. Soon they passed through the city gates. Before them tree-lined boulevards opened onto bountiful markets filled with fabric shops, tea houses, and food stalls. Beyond, there were quiet gardens, libraries, temples, colleges, and fine residences. Warm breezes carried the scent of spices, perfumes, the faint sounds of chanting. The voyagers were overcome with wonder. The residents welcomed the travelers as long-lost kinsmen, and found food and lodging for them. In the coming months, the voyagers rested. Many took advantage of the rich spiritual life there; they found teachers, they studied, debated, and meditated.

Finally, the guide saw that his band of seekers had regained their strength and confidence. Early one morning, while they were all asleep, he dissolved the splendid city into thin air. Suddenly, they all woke up to find themselves on bare rocky ground. Nothing remained of their previous comforts. There was nothing but a cold cloudless blue sky, harsh mountains, and a rocky pathway. The followers looked around in shock. Indeed, they felt they were waking from a dream.

The guide explained: "The city you thought you were visiting was a phantom place I conjured by weaving together the strands of your longings and desires. It was an illusion I produced to restore your strength of body and clarity of mind. We must now go on to find the treasure you set out to seek. It is very near."

This is a famous story told in many places, most notably in the Lotus Sutra. There, the guide is not identified as a Buddha, but he is said to be someone who faces the similar problem of encouraging seekers to continue on the harsh path to liberation. Perhaps he is a Bodhisattva, perhaps some other kind of wise person. But no matter which telling one encounters, this parable is puzzling. At the center of our puzzlement is the nature of the conjured city.

The sutra says that within the city, the seekers "feel they have been saved from their difficulties, they have a complete sense of ease and tranquility." This place then is something more profound than a pleasant spa. The description makes the city seem like a modest version of what they are already searching for. It is a refuge from the demands of a much harsher world. It provides a structure in which "ease and tranquility" can be cultivated, and a context in which the seeker can be "saved." From this point of view, the conjured city appears to mirror the edifice of the Buddha's teachings. It is a realm where awareness is cultivated in the format of teachings, teachers, and students.

The conjured city is a temporary illusion that the guide produces to enable seekers to clarify their sense of goal and strengthen their resolve to reach it. It is an illusion which produces healing. It is an illusion that brings clarity, even wisdom. It is a structure that the guide, here representing the Buddha, creates and then makes disappear. The seekers must return to the world if they are themselves to become capable of holding the treasures that alleviate suffering, impoverishment, and confusion in all humankind. When the guide has dispersed the entire conjured city back into nothingness, he tells the seekers that the treasure they seek is now near and they must go on.

The seekers have, without the slightest warning, been stripped of the comforts and routines from which they had been benefitting. They have been dumped onto a cold and rocky road. That's the end of the story. It doesn't tell us whether they were shocked, outraged at the guide's deception, or questioned their faith because of his manipulation. We assume not. We accept that the strength the seekers re-awakened during their sojourn in illusion, even when revealed as such, has enabled them to continue. They are like newborn children in a world that is bright and uncomfortable, hard and freezing cold, but at the same time they know that what they yearn for is not dependent on the dream-forms in which they gained their insight and strength.

Indeed, it may be, as centuries later, Marcel Proust would marvel:

"Perhaps it is not-being that is the true state, and all our dream of life is inexistent, but if so, we feel that phrases of music, conceptions which exist in relation to our dream must be nothing either. We shall perish, but we have as hostages these divine captives who will follow and share our fate. And death in their company is somehow less bitter, less inglorious, perhaps even less probable."

II

As has been said repeatedly: mind itself is intrinsically unstable. Traditionally, mind has been described as "that which seeks an object." In other words, it is in the nature of mind to be forever seeking, forever on the move between a subjective pole, a kind of self, and an objective pole, something designated other. This bouncing back and forth process is unending. Should we adjust ourselves, our attitudes and outlooks? Should we move more decisively to obtain what we want from the world? Such problems are compounded because we know that our sense of our identity is always shifting; our intellectual and emotional frameworks are in flux; navigating between our changing desires and the changing outer world, we must always find new channels, sea lanes, new compass points.

This is always the case, but right now, our insecurity seems even more intense. The world, our assumptions about the world and our place in it, seem to be shaking apart. Certainty and the means of reaching it have also been shaken. The materialistic outlook, the belief that we should bend our minds and our world to fit our goals, has led to inner and outer catastrophe. There are innumerable possibilities. There is a strange atmospheric silence. We feel vulnerable in unsuspected ways. We feel chaos closing in. Our memories are not helpful. It is all as painful and uncertain and unstoppable as being born anew.

The 13th-century Zen Master Dogen Zenji said:

> "Birth is just like riding in a boat. You raise the sails and row with the oar. Although you row, the boat gives you the ride, and without the boat, no one could ride. But you ride in the boat and your riding makes the boat what it is. Investigate a moment such as this.

> "At just such a moment, there is nothing but the world of the boat. The sky, the water, and the shore are all the boat's world, which is not the same as a world that is not the boat's.

> "When you ride in a boat, your body and mind and the environs together are the undivided activity of the boat. The entire earth and the entire sky are both the undivided activity of the boat. Thus birth is nothing but you; you are nothing but birth."

But how to find our way? All the forebears of all Buddhist lineage tell us simply to look at our own mind. Look at the space in which movement arises, remains, dies. Look at the mind, look as thoughts, emotions, ideas come, go, link. That is the basis of everything, inner or outer, of what we understand and experience, and what we accomplish.

To look at the mind while not following thoughts, that is the path. In the Buddhist tradition there are innumerable kinds of practice and meditation, but all are inseparable from this. The path moves from being conditioned by goals into dimensions of unconditioned freedom. It concludes in acknowledging compassion, the spontaneous conjunctions of our innumerable realities. We move amid innumerable journeys. Whatever is called enlightenment, compassion, ego, wakefulness, practice, kindness, meditation, mind, Buddha. These seem to be nouns, but really they are vectors, momentary forms of motion, colors of light. They weave us in and out of the world and time. Stopping, and certainty they are momentary.

We journey and continue seeking as the inhabitants of an empty boat. And we are the conveyance for others.

Dogen Zenji said: "Know that there are innumerable beings in yourself."

In early summer evenings, beneath the mulberry tree at the foot of the garden, fireflies flickered an otherworldly neon green in the humid lavender dark. I was five, and on one special night my sisters, my brother, and I were allowed to go out into the dusk and catch fireflies. Our mother gave us jars with holes poked in the top, and we ran barefoot beneath the trees, catching the small fluorescent creatures as fallen berries in the grass squelched beneath our feet.

By morning light we could see that many fireflies in the jar had died, and that those living were shabby grayish bugs. But now we saw our feet were dyed a wonderful shade of purple-blue.

§ § §

Not far from the museum, without realizing where I had strayed, I found myself looking at the familiar Art Deco façade of an apartment building where two friends had lived long ago. They had been very old when I knew them. The wife had lived much longer, and I'd always felt guilty because I put off visiting her. Lolya was small, bitter, tremulous, angry, pale, bulldog-like, and usually half-drunk. In her late teens, in 1920, she had managed to escape Russia. The Bolsheviks had just *about solidified their grip. There was no place for the daughter of a governor-general, a princess. Her parents had been killed. Her life was harsh. Now, she'd been in New York a long time, taught history of science, art, worked as a social worker, and later an archivist. Her husband had been a fixture in the New York art world, maintained by marginal academic positions. Recently he'd lost his mind, insisting he would soon join a group of young poets from his native Greece on the shores of the Black Sea. She put him in a nursing home where he lingered in confusion and sorrow. She was disgusted with him and wouldn't visit. She'd relied on me to see him, report back on his condition. He died fairly soon.*

Still, I made myself visit. As usual, she offered me tea in an unclean cup while she drank cheap scotch, smoked Pall Malls, and in her yeasty Russian accent, she liked to lecture.

She held up her fingers one by one: "One, ownership, including slavery; Two, hierarchical order; Three, war; these are the things in human society that never, never change. Read history. It's true. No one wants to admit it." She closed her eyes, then opened them and stared at me. "You disagree? Whatever you think is good, your literature, your art, your music, your religion, whatever, it only exists to hide the need to possess, to dominate, to destroy." She gazed out the window at the pale sky. She shook her head. "You have no idea." A long pause followed.

"You really think so?" I asked cautiously.

"I'm not sure where thinking fits in. Why thinking? Why thinking at all? It's a trap." She slugged down the last of the whiskey. Her eyes watered. She glanced at a picture of her husband on the side-table. "You know, I never should have married him."

————A VANISHED SAGE:
BIDYA DANDARON

B idya Dandaron was born in Kizhinga, Buryatia on December 28, 1914. His mother was a dedicated Buddhist practitioner, the widow of a wandering lama, Dazarof Dandar. His stepfather was Dorje Badmaev, the closest student and Dharma heir of the renowned Lubsan Samdan Tsydenov, sometime-abbot of Kudun Datsan, a holder of both Gelugpa and Nyingma lineages. Dandaron's stepfather began teaching him from earliest childhood. When he was three, a party of Gelugpa monks from Tibet came to inform Dandaron's family that their son had been recognized as the reincarnation of Jayagsy Rinpoche, Tsydenov's teacher and the abbot of Kumbum Monastery in Tibet. They wished to take him to Tibet for training, but Tsydenov and his father felt that it was better for the boy to stay in Buryatia. The monks departed; monastic officials later recognized an alternative candidate.

Dandaron continued to live and study with his parents in Soorkhoi where a small community of practitioners lived under Tsydenov's auspices. During this time, a number of armies, some little more than bandit gangs, criss-crossed Siberia and the Mongolian steppes, each trying to secure its own base to resist the Red Armies taking over Russia.

In 1919, in an effort to help 13,000 Buryatia who had requested his protection, Tsydenov took the extraordinary step of proclaiming a Buddhist kingdom where he, as a Cakravartin or Dharmaraja, ruled. His government contained strong Western influences. A constituent assembly was elected by popular vote, and all the government ministers were elected from that body. All laws were made in accord with Buddhist doctrine; non-violence was the law of the land, and all Buryatia were exempt from being drafted into any of the surrounding armies.

Tsydenov, despite the death of his successor Badmaev in 1919, was able to maintain this kingdom for a year. Then he was taken prisoner by Ataman Grigory Semyonov's agents and moved further into northern Siberia. In 1921, during a public ceremony at a small temple in Sholuta, Tsydenov proclaimed that Bidya Dandaron was his successor as Dharmaraja. Soon after, the Soviets captured Tsydenov, and he was never seen again.

D andaron was seven when Tsydenov left, but he did not forget him, though he never pursued claims to Tsydenov's title. It seems that he and his mother moved to Khyagta, a small city three hours south of Ulan-Ude, the Buryat capital. Dandaron would continue Buddhist study and practice there, and at the same time attended the state high school where mathematics, sciences and, of course, Communist doctrine made up a great deal of the curriculum. And how proud his teachers must have been that someone with such a primitive background was capable of mastering the languages and scientific knowledge needed for acceptance into the Aircraft Device Construction

Institute in Leningrad, where he studied aeronautical engineering from 1934 to 1937.

During this time, he got married and had two children. He also audited classes in Tibetan at the Oriental Studies Institute of the Leningrad State University. The depth of his understanding and experience in Buddhist teachings, as well as his openness to Western analytical methods, made a great impression on many of the students and faculty members. He deepened his study of the Tibetan language with Andrei Vostrikov, with whom he became particularly close.

At the end of 1937, towards the conclusion of the great wave of Stalinist purges, Dandaron was arrested as a spy for Japan and an agent of an alleged "pan-Mongolian Conspiracy." This was part of the Soviet's unrelenting effort to erase any religion which could be a focus for nationalist sentiment.

Shortly after Dandaron's arrest, Vostrikov was taken into custody and executed. Dandaron was sentenced to a six-year term of hard labor at a camp in Siberia. His wife and children were allowed to accompany him, but left after several months. His wife contracted pneumonia and died, as did one of the children.

Labor camps in the vast Gulag all required that days be spent in heavy manual work such as mining, road construction, ditch digging, and forestry. The weather conditions were extreme. By night, prisoners were packed into bunks in wooden dormitories. The stench was overwhelming. Rations were barely edible, calculated to keep prisoners on the edge of starvation. There was no sanitation to speak of. Discipline was arbitrary and brutal. Violence was continuous. Death rates were, as intended, high.

As one survivor explained: "The Gulag was conceived in order to transform human matter into a docile, exhausted, ill-smelling mass…thinking of nothing but how to appease the constant torture of hunger, living in the instant, concerned with nothing apart from evading kicks, cold, and ill treatment. ...All human emotions — love, friendship, envy, concern for one's fellow man, compassion, longing for fame, honesty — had left us with the flesh that had melted from our bodies..."

Dandaron lived in these conditions for six years. He was often tortured, and forever after bore the scars inflicted by the back of a Cossack's sabre. Nonetheless, he found ways to continue meditative and yogic practice. He was also able to continue studying books that were smuggled in to him, to send and receive an occasional letter, and to teach fellow inmates ways of meditating that adapted to the extreme nature of this situation. He was released in 1943.

The next five years were marked by a momentary softening in the government's attitude towards religions. Ivolginsky and Aginsky monasteries were re-opened under the supervision of government agencies, but "wandering lamas" taught and performed ceremonies privately. Dandaron was able to renew some of his former friendships in both Leningrad and Ulan-Ude. He resumed translating texts. Small groups of Western and Buryat practitioners began meeting with him.

But Dandaron was again arrested in 1947 and given a ten-year sentence as part of renewed anti-religious purges. The conditions of his imprisonment in Ulan-Ude were evidently not as harsh as his earlier confinement. He also benefited from the companionship of some Buryat lamas and Western philosophers who had been swept into the government's net. He considered himself particularly lucky to be able to study Kant with the Lithuanian philosopher Vasily Seseman. He became increasingly interested in the conjunction of Western and Buddhist thought. He was also able to write a wide range of articles and commentaries, but most of these were intercepted and destroyed.

Dandaron now attracted disciples from Buryatia, Russia, Ukraine, Latvia, and Estonia, many highly educated in a wide range of subjects. These fellow prisoners became his most loyal adherents and became what was later called the core of the "Sangha of Dandaron." He taught what he called "neo-Buddhism" in which he explored combining Buddhism with European philosophy and science.

His group viewed practice and study not as an exterior preoccupation, but as an exploration of the inner ways in which Buddhist practice and thought illuminated, and were illuminated by, their lives in the labor camp. It was, as Dandaron called it, the "collective Karma" they shared with the Soviet world as a whole.

In February of 1956, Nikita Khrushchev gave his famous speech to the Communist Party Congress in Moscow in which he repudiated the excesses of Stalin's cult of personality in general, and, more specifically, the mass imprisonments in the Gulag. Within a year, Dandaron found himself rehabilitated and released.

He joked that "for a Buddhist journeying from one incarnation to another, it was very useful to be born in Russia." He added, laughing: "Note that I say Buddhist and not Buddhists."

In 1957, he renewed his contacts in Leningrad, but friends and colleagues were unable to find him a permanent position there. Dandaron was, however, able to find work at the Buryat Institute of Social Sciences in Ulan-Ude. There he worked with three other Buryat lamas on cataloguing and overseeing the preservation of the large number of books that had formerly been part of monastic libraries, most notably on the Tibetan Kanjur (collected sutras) and Tenjur (commentaries). He traveled frequently to Leningrad, and there, by a stroke of luck, met George Roerich, son of the famous painter and theosophical philosopher. Roerich was, in his own right, a great and widely traveled Tibetologist, and the two began working closely together, producing a large number of scholarly papers. Among Dandaron's papers were: "The Buddhist Theory of the Individual 'I', " "Contents of the Mantra Om-ma-ni-pad-me-hum," and an article for the Russian Encyclopedia of Buddhism on the Aga Monastery. It was a great blow, both to Dandaron and to Buddhist studies in Russia, when Roerich died suddenly in 1960. Nonetheless, Dandaron continued to produce studies on Buddhist religion and history, as well as Tibetan-Russian translations of Buddhist texts. He also wrote essays exploring ways in which Buddhist conceptions could enrich and develop Western philosophical and scientific thought, and reciprocally how Western thinking could find a place in the continuum of classical Buddhist concerns. These were distributed via samizdat.

At the same time, a group of students, some formerly from the camps, others from the academic world, began to gather around him. Sometimes he would go to Leningrad, and sometimes the students would take the week-long train ride to Ulan-Ude. As Dandaron said: "It's not that students are coming to me in Ulan-Ude; it's Buddhism that is moving westward."

His tantric teaching at this time was focused on the practice of Yamantaka, Conqueror of the Lord of Death. Though these have always been secret teachings, it seems that Dandaron emphasized the approach in which all the bardos, all the transitions in life, dream, meditation, death, and rebirth, all the unending transitions in what we call existence and non-existence, each and every one is the path of enlightenment.

In a series talks published in Moscow in 1970, Dandaron began: "Our knowledge is limited by the boundaries of Samsara and by the manifestation of Nirvana (each of which) has its own limits, namely, the limits of our system of time and space and the physical world order in which we move. About such knowledge in any other time or era, we must admit that substance and character are unknown to us."

"Buddhism," he said, "has neither place nor time nor epoch. Buddhism journeys on, unaware of peoples, countries, climates, revivals or declines, societies or social groups. This does not mean that Buddhism denies such things. Buddhism denies nothing. This means that Buddhism itself is not aware of them. Such things are not its concern."

"Dandaron is bodhisattva-mahasattva. He is a hero," said his student Vladimir Montlevich. "He was unburdened by the horizons of dogma. He tore that away. He also intuited the needs of our time, and, in this, he was exactly as he said: 'a Neo-Buddhist'."

D andaron had always been viewed with suspicion and dislike by members of the Buryat Communist apparatus in Ulan-Ude. He upheld traditions that they wanted to leave behind in their effort to find a modern identity. They expected him to show the Russians that people of the steppes were as capable as anyone of contributing to modern communism. But he had betrayed them. Late one night, young Buryat communists destroyed the stupas he and his followers had built in honor of his teacher, Samdan Tsydenov, and his stepfather, Dorje Badmaev. No doubt, they were at the bottom of the denunciations that led to Dandaron's arrest and the charges that were laid against him when he was arrested in Leningrad in 1972.

On December 27, 1972, Dandaron was tried in Ulan-Ude under Article 227 of the Soviet Criminal Code. He was accused of leading a Buddhist sect that participated in "bloody sacrifices" and "ritual copulations" and of attempting to "murder or beat former members of the sect who wanted to leave it." Further charges included "contacts with foreign countries and international Zionism." Finally, most charges were dropped, but the contentions that the "Dandaron Group" held prayer meetings, had an illicit financial fund, and that Mr. Dandaron acted as 'guru' to the group, were accepted without proof. Four associates, Yuri K. Lavrov, the painter Alexei Zheleznov, D.

Butkus, and the philosopher V. M. Montlevich, were subjected to psychological examination, found mentally ill, and sent to psychiatric institutions from which they were soon released. Dandaron was handed a sentence of five years deprivation of freedom under conditions of forced labor in a corrective labor colony at Vydrino, on the southern shore of Lake Baikal. Despite his age and failing health, he was required to do hard labor.

"Oh the wonder of Vajrasattva," Bidya Dandarovich Dandaron exclaimed. Not quite sixty, with a broken arm and his leg barely healed, he was forced back onto a work gang. He was still teaching people who came to him in secret, and these students took great risks to smuggle in food to sustain him. He was a scholar renowned for his mastery of Buddhist and Western philosophy, but the world of monasteries, monks, and renowned teachers was completely gone. He now taught a path of Buddhist tantric practice entirely adapted to the brutality of the age.

In the bleak and unending life of the camps, a world devoid of comfort, privacy, silence, consolation, or future, stranded in an expanse of hardened mud, dry grass, and impassible forests, beneath a horizonless sky of roiling gray clouds, Dandaron proclaimed the name of Vajrasattva. He was allowed an occasional visitor. It was said that for those who heard him directly, the effect was of a sudden clap of thunder, a bolt of lightning, a sudden opening in the sky. Some reported that those who did not hear him directly sensed a momentary, almost painful joy, a near but not quite accessible bright expanse, hidden within clouds and beneath the plains.

At that point, Dandaron recognized that all Vajrayana practices could be explored in the single deity of Vajrasattva. He evolved a method of practice with a purifying aspect, and added a complex visualization with an outer form and inner mandala. These were the intrinsic forms of all-pervasive radiance that extended through all of space to dissipate the ignorance and suffering of every living being. At times, Dandaron would sit unmoving as his breathing and his heartbeat would stop. In late 1973, he fell and broke an arm and leg. He was forced to return to work before they were healed. He spoke of wanting to build a round white temple to Vajrasattva on his release. Dandaron said: "I unite all schools."

On October 26, 1974, at the age of sixty, he said: "The Dakinis (female emanations of wisdom) are calling to me." Again he went into a long meditative trance. His heart and breathing stopped. He sat motionless for a long time, but did not return to this life. The prison authorities would not say where his body had been buried.

Here
Radiant skies of Compassion
Shine
Without thought.

Look:
Before space opens
Hear:
Before time begins

Leap

Into the Diamond Heart
Vajrasattva
Present
Everywhere.

And hallucinations
Of the world's pain and terror,
The world's longing
Whirl, vanish slowly in the sky.

Just two weeks before Dandaron's death, the painter Andrei I. Zheleznov, an early student of Dandaron's and one who had been convicted in the same trial as he, completed a thangka painting of the mandala of Yamantaka, Conqueror of Death. The mandala itself is a traditional presentation. In its center, Yamantaka, wrathful and with the head of a water buffalo, stands surrounded by his retinue in the pure land of his attributes and powers. Around them are the lineage of deities and teachers who have transmitted the outer and inner meaning of this great wrathful one.

But in Zheleznov's painting, within the outer precincts of the palace, are depictions of all those people most important to Dandaron: his step-father Dorje Badmaev, two images of his teacher Samdan Tsydenov (one wearing humble robes, the other dressed in the ornaments of a Cakravartin), and a portrait of Lama Jayagsy. Outside the mandala, among other deities and teachers, Dandaron himself is portrayed in his roles of yogi, teacher, and lineage holder. He wears prison garb, a suit, and a deity's crown and ornaments. This, then, is how Dandaron's disciples finally saw him, and practiced as they followed him: passing through suffering and death, passing from life to life, invincible, indestructible love, and endlessly wakening.

§ § §

In Halifax, Nova Scotia, in the late fall of 1986, The Vidyadhara, Chögyam Trungpa Rinpoche, a great pioneer in bringing the Buddhist teachings from Tibet to the West, had a catastrophic heart attack. This caused a collapse of his liver functions, and, until his death on April 4, 1987, he suffered a long sequence of heart and organ failures, and regular hospitalizations with near-death episodes. But after the first collapse I sat by his bed in the intensive care unit as the artificial lung machine wheezed and thumped. There was no way, I thought, that a human body can withstand this. I knew that with his death a large part of my life would soon be at an end. What would follow, I, like all of his other students, could not imagine. But an unknowable transformation was looming, and could not be escaped.

I visited Rinpoche about once a month for the next half-year. At first he tried to speak, made kinds of grunts, then simply looked and exhaled. He scratched himself, then barely moved. It was clear that, month by month, he was fading. But to those who attended him every day, this was not perceptible. They issued optimistic bulletins about how he would resume his teaching schedule. They did this not out of a desire to deceive, but simply because they could not countenance the losses on a daily basis. Rinpoche and those caring for him lived together in a large house where everything was centered on Rinpoche's continued existence, and to think otherwise was beyond disloyalty. They created around him an atmosphere of determined possessiveness. They would never let him go.

In the midst of this, Rinpoche himself was no longer capable of normal communication. And yet, and yet, he was intensely present, attentive, waiting. The first time I visited, it was shocking. Seated, strapped into his chair, his face was rigid, strangely transformed. But then I felt a poignant autumnal pale-gold afternoon light. I looked at him, his ravaged physiology, and I felt a harsh pang of grief, but around this depth of loss was something clear, gentle, unwavering.

Nurses and technicians, people who were not his students and had never known him when he was active, also found themselves deeply moved. Each time I visited, the atmosphere around him shifted like the light of a waning sun. But the light was not dimming. It was a different shade of dark gold, then lavender, lavender deep purple.

The last time I saw Trungpa Rinpoche alive, he was again in the hospital. I glimpsed into the hospital room. He was lying on his side, gazing at his wife who sat at the bedside. There was a feeling of waiting to depart, of waiting by a gate in moonlight. Romantic, sad, continuing in his love for her, his love for this inconstant and painful world.

————FOR MUSIC

… in an instant of awareness,
Infinite Buddhas,
Simultaneous shining
Everywhere interrelated:

A vast humming.
… the ocean of Buddhas;
…the mind of enlightenment.
…harmonies
heard beyond hearing

Waves of delirium
Absorbing all distinctions.

The vector of finding or grasping or attaining or knowing;
This is a core of movement we cannot imagine absent:
This gives us the sense of what is next or falling away or
    lost or unattainable.

A desire, a fear divides a world,
A focus divides a mind,
A purpose creates our refuse,

In the surrounding moment,
A world, a range of things sensed or to be sensed:
Horizons shimmer.
We expand and contract

A student took the renowned Tibetan teacher Rabjam Rinpoch, to hear a concert of Western classical symphonic music. At the end, Rinpoche asked: "Do you listen to this music horizontally or vertically?"

Night Rain at Kuang-k'ou
by Yang Wan-Li

The river is clear and calm;
a fast rain falls in the gorge.
At midnight the cold, splashing sound begins,
like thousands of pearls spilling onto a glass plate,
each drop penetrating the bone.
In my dream I scratch my head and get up to listen.
I listen and listen, until the dawn.
All my life I have heard rain,
and I am an old man;
but now for the first time I understand
the sound of spring rain
on the river at night.

Nine hundred years ago, Yang dreamed he woke as a storm broke around him on the river where his boat was anchored. But unsure of whether he was dreaming or awake, he listened, and a new understanding of rain came to him. Now, here, miraculously beyond such concepts as awake or dream, now or then, Yang gives us the presence of that moment again, and with it he shares a sense of sound not constrained by space and time. So simple, so complex. Even if we may be clinging to a single mind-stream, a single self, there are so many strands in this instant.

Polyphony, deploying many voices simultaneously, is perhaps the most extraordinary characteristic of Western classical music. Notated scores have made the extensive development of highly complex polyphonic music possible. And so we have a long tradition that continually finds new life in complex sound structures. As members of the audience, we listen not just for a melody or a rhythm, but we strive to open our ears to hear all the notes, all the rhythms, all the balances and dynamics within an evolving aural architecture that rises and vanishes in time.

"Gerald de Barri, a 12th-century Welsh churchman writing as Giraldus Cambrensis, made a famous description of his peasant countrymen's communal singing: 'They sing their tunes not in unison, but in parts with many simultaneous modes and phrases. Therefore, in a group of singers you will hear as many melodies as you will see heads, yet they all accord in one consonant and properly constituted composition.' "

This sensibility has also enriched our literature. Mikhail Bakhtin discussed the polyphonic aspects of Rabelais' writing, and in his celebrated study of Dostoevsky, described literary polyphony as occurring when: "the voices remain independent and, as such are combined in a unity of a higher order... (thus) a combination of several individual wills takes place, (so) that the boundaries of the individual will can be in principle exceeded."

This kind of attention lets us listen to not just one sequence of sounds or words, but several simultaneously. We follow interweaving melodies and thoughts, and find ourselves also in the unsuspected spaces between them. And there emerges a kind of sound (or language) architecture as notes (or written words) dissolve and others begin, then remain in the air for differing extents of time. Composers, performers, and authors give us passage into these structures, and we, the audience, join together as we explore them.

The natural expanse,
Free from seeking, cultivation, definitions,

Receives the awakened state
As a mountain receives the light of the sun, moon, and stars,
Receives blankets of snows,
Receives torrents of rain from clouds,
Receives the lifecycles of insects, worms, germs, birds, foxes,
     wolves, beetles,
Receives cold winds, spring breezes in oak, cedar, pine,
     maple, brushwood,
Receives cascades of melting water,
Receives avalanches of rocks,
Receives fire,
Receives hunters, pilgrims, merchants, lovers on the run.

Allowing goals to determine how we cultivate mind radically reduces the expanse, quality, and depth, as well as overall movement of what we understand, feel, see, know, share, etc. Choosing actions solely on the basis of their intended outcome is the root of our ecological catastrophe.

How crucial then to attend to the random, the puzzling, the strangely beautiful, the unforeseen, the irrelevant, the rejected, the peripheral, the ever elusive, the flirty, the unconnected, the gap. How crucial to know that we cannot possess our experience.

Anna Lowenhaupt Tsing's *The Mushroom at the End of The World* is an extraordinary, complex, and beautifully written book focused on matsutake mushrooms. This fungus, cherished and prized by Japanese and Koreans because its scent evokes the sadness of the end of autumn, grows only in devastated landscapes, particularly in the over-logged forests of Oregon. There they are harvested commercially by US Army vets seeking "freedom," former Thai soldiers and Cambodian refugees, as well as old Japanese people for whom the mushroom and hunting brings back the folkways demolished when their families were put in concentration camps here. The book's subtitle is "On The Possibility of Life in Capitalist Ruins."

Dr. Tsing writes of the complex biologies, histories, economies, and ecologies that intertwine in the matsutake mushrooms' life, environment, value, harvesting. As she says: "Many histories come together here: they draw us beyond bubble worlds into shifting cascades of collaboration and complexity…rather than limiting our analyses to one creature at a time (including humans), or even one relationship, if we want to know what makes places livable we should be studying the polyphonic assemblages, gatherings of ways of being. Assemblages are performances of livability."

The anthropologist Eduardo Kohn has written on how forests can be said to "think" since, within the jungle, the interplay of phenomena from the atmospheric, geological, biological, animal, and human realms are continually influencing each other, and in this way are producing a multiplicity of continuously unfolding meanings of these phenomena. Thus the forest is recognizably a mind, if not an exclusively human one. That is to say, its shifting forms of organization and awareness are not exclusively devoted to human purposes.

"Selves," Kohn says, speaking of human and non-human beings in his study of the Runa of the upper Amazon, "exist simultaneously as embodied and beyond the body. They are localized and yet they exceed the individual and even the human…"

"This spirit realm that emerges from the life of the forest, as a product of a whole host of relations that cross species lines and temporal epochs, is, then, a zone of continuity and possibility… survival depends on many kinds of deaths that this spirit realm holds in its configuration and that make a living future possible."

So, there is an infinite unfolding of musical sequences in innumerable simultaneous dimensions. We, in our speaking, singing, thinking, crying, laughing are ourselves living sequences of sound. Our attention, our hearing, our waiting, our silence extend the space in which sound is moving.

Each tone moves through time with its qualities: pitch, shifting dynamics, evolving colors, altering relationship with pitches before, after, above, below, near or far, and/or simultaneously. By the shift of relationship, each pitch is heard differently, and the spatial environment changes.

No pitch has its own unique history or fate. There is only the simultaneous and evolving multiplicity.

Such a complex and informative array of sound is not just a human artifact. Bernie Krause is a musician and acoustician who has spent the last fifty years recording the soundscapes of diverse natural environments all over the world. Patiently, he has listened to and recorded the rich and various polyphony of pine forests, jungles, seashores, deserts, swamps, rivers, open plains, alpine mountains. As he tells, the first time he began recording such an environment, "the captured ambiences — rich textures that infused the entire frequency spectrum with elegant structures, multiple tempi and soloists — intensified my experience of the habitat through their luxurious and subtle nuances." All our music, from the simplest to the most complicated, has emerged from this ravishing and splendid display. Krause has made many thousands of such recordings which now, when he has returned to sites whose sound-life he formerly recorded, show a deepening sterile silence, the devastating effects of human interventions of innumerable kinds.

Recently this may have become more vivid to us, as the pandemic and radically decreased economic activity brought a halt to airplane, truck, and automobile traffic. Birds long silent were bright and audible; racoons, foxes, coyotes sang at dusk. This was a fertile quiet, slightly disconcerting but calling to us in a deep way we had not quite forgotten. Listening, it seems, could carry us further. And now, even as traffic returns, the older stillness haunts us; makes us uneasy. Silence and the sounds from realms that are not ours are only hiding; we are waiting for their return.

Were we to explore without stopping, would it be possible for us to hear, to recognize as the sage Nagarjuna did so long ago, that "wandering in the pain of this cyclical illusion has nothing that distinguishes it from liberation. Liberation has nothing that distinguishes it from wandering in the pain of this cyclical illusion."

It has begun, almost without noticing,
It seems sudden:
Time, so laboriously expended,
Vanishes.
A day is gone.

And, somehow, effort was expended to no end.
The sought-for transformation vanishes.
And so, at the end — evening:

What is being called "I" changes and doesn't.
The world surrounding moves beyond its own
Thunderstorm, stop; sunburst, stop; light rain and the dense
smell of green and trees,
Sounds of waking women, men,
Scents of soap, of burning wood, coffee:
The unsought passage.
Bells, pigeons clattering in flight,
Dream and awake
Wave on wave:
Unending and unbegun
Weaving
Music

Thank you.

In memory of Peter Serkin

THE NOBLE HEART OF EXISTENCE

In most of human history, people have lived in small communities among those with whom they had lifelong associations and intimacies. Distant plagues, mass starvation in foreign countries, wars in far-off lands, even destruction of unfamiliar civilizations — all these events passed by, unknown to those who were remote from them.

Today we live in transient groupings among people we have met only recently, if at all. But internet and television make us vividly aware of the many forms of suffering everywhere on the globe. Hourly we see the bloody faces of the casualties of war, the wracked and wasted bodies of starving children, the cries and tears of the murder victim's family. These images of suffering around the world are often more familiar to us than the gravest difficulties of our neighbors, even as social media presents the most private kinds of desperation and pain of people we scarcely know.

Increasingly, as the distant face of suffering becomes more intimate, our isolation becomes more intense. But now we share our loneliness and helplessness on a global scale. Our immediate longing to relieve the pain of those we encounter on television or the internet becomes our own desire for relief, and we are locked together in an encompassing experience of frustration.

As our helplessness drifts into apathy and then a weary resentment, we look for ways to distance ourselves from the pain and suffering that crowd around us. Our own needs are going unmet. Why can't those other people help themselves? Aren't they, in one way or another, the cause of their own misery? And so we come to see the victims as members of a mindlessly aggressive society, or of a culture irretrievably attached to faulty agricultural methods, or of an ethnic group that simply won't sustain normal family patterns. If only they would move, get an education, or somehow just disappear.

Surrounded by continuous violence, destruction, sickness, we feel burdened by caring and resentful of our innate sympathies. In such circumstances, the experience of compassion as real and available becomes deformed, and confidence in the power of compassion fades.

In ordinary usage, according to the OED, "compassion" means first: "suffering together with another, participation in suffering; fellow feeling, sympathy," and second: "the feeling or emotion as moved by the distress of another and the desire to relieve it." Buddhism, however, understands compassion as something far more extensive than merely a feeling or emotion, with all the itinerant qualities which those words imply.

The Vajrayana Buddhist tradition of Tibet maintains that the complete and entire basis of our life in this world is compassion. According to this view:

In the infinite expanse of the natural state
Free from the limits of conceptual mind,
All the realms of life and death and their inhabitants
Arise spontaneously from the radiance of Great Compassion.

The Tibetan word for compassion, *nyingje*, literally means "noble heart," and this refers not simply to one's own heart, but to the heart of the world as well. It is called "heart" because compassion is at the core of all our responses to external and internal phenomena. It is the basis of why our minds always move outside ourselves, why our perceptions lead us out into the world of phenomena, and why we are spontaneously moved by the sight of beauty and suffering, the smell of early spring or rotting garbage, the memory of the taste of lemonade, the sound of thunder in the afternoon.

Compassion is mind's innate movement outward. It is the underlying momentum of our emotional and perceptual experience. If we examine even our most self-absorbed thought, we always find it is prompted by the vivid awareness of something we consider outside ourselves. Even when we are concerned with pain in our own body, that pain is somehow viewed as "other," as something alien to our "real" self. In fact, no matter what the emotional twist, all our thoughts begin with the sense of "other." So, at the core, our heart places others before ourselves. Thus, because our mind is naturally inclined to concern with others, it is called "noble."

At the center of all our mental functioning, as the natural basis of all our perceptions, instincts, impulses, and more elaborated motivations, is this primordial awareness of other, this "noble heart."

Tibetan Buddhist traditions describe three aspects to the experience of compassion:

1) There is compassion as occasioned by awareness of the specific suffering and pain of others.

2) There is compassion arising from awareness of the inescapable causes of suffering.

3) There is compassion without reference point, free, omnipresent, ever-expanding and continuous.

One afternoon, I sat with my wife's colleague and friend Iván in a Budapest bakery renowned for flódni, a confection with layers of poppy seed, walnut, and apple. We were in the old Jewish neighborhood only a few blocks from the Great Synagogue.

"You see that door over there?" He pointed a thick hand at a faded green door across the street which, no doubt, gave onto an interior courtyard. I turned and peered. There was nothing special about it.

"Yes."

"My cousin, Tomi, you know him?"

"Yes, we spent last night wandering all along the river with him." Iván's cousin was a retired chemical engineer, a great connoisseur of all kinds of local history, and a delight to wander with though the city.

"Well, you know that shit Eichmann, just a few months before the war ended, rounded up all the Jews." I nodded. "He loaded them in barges on the Danube to take them to Auschwitz. And they were all herded along this street right out front."

"Ah."

"Tomi and all his family were in the crowd being pushed down the street. And someone opened that door and suddenly grabbed them, told them to shut up, pulled them into the courtyard. That's why they lived. Tomi, all of them. They risked their lives, the people who saved them." I shook my head. "And you know what? We never knew who those people were, and we never found out."

And it seemed, at that moment, that what Iván was telling me was not so much a Holocaust story, or a Jewish story, or even a family story; he was showing something miraculous woven into the fabric of an ordinary street.

§ § §

Generally, our most direct experience of compassion is occasioned by the awareness of suffering itself. When we hear of the illness of someone we love, when we see a wounded animal, and even when we hear of someone whom we despise suffering the loss of a child, we feel that pain well up in our heart. Here we experience the utter spontaneity of compassion, which rises up past all distinctions and differences, predilections and conceptual frameworks.

However, our habitual second thought, particularly with respect to those who are not close to us, is to draw away from the sight of others' suffering, just as we try to distance ourselves from our own experience of pain. Just as we feel isolated within our own pain, we tend to isolate others in theirs. In doing so, we tend to justify ourselves by referring to a body of conventional concepts and secret fears; we try to secure our own "needs" and "preserve our boundaries."

But no matter what conceptualizations we may make use of in these circumstances, we cannot quite ignore that this life is filled with disappointments, sorrow, sickness, death, and continuous sufferings of many kinds. Suffering is universal and unavoidable. This cannot be escaped, no matter how we invoke the decency of our aspirations, the excellence of our successes, the virtue of our goals, or the reality of our powerlessness.

We can cut through the morass of reflexive ego-clinging in many ways, but the essence of how to do so is always the same: we put the needs and concerns of others before our own. This is practiced in simple acts of courtesy, as well as in many kinds of attention, generosity, care, and consideration. Parents routinely put the lives and aspirations of their children ahead of their own satisfactions; people often make sacrifices to take care of parents and friends. These kinds of actions, which go on continuously and unremarked, are the essence of social life. Acting in this way, we constantly discover that we do not need to rely on compulsive ego-centered logic. There is a vast range of possibilities alive right before us, revealed in the light of how we take care of the world around us.

Compassion that is occasioned by suffering itself brings us into this world ever more fully. We cannot escape what arises in our hearts, even if we are unable to prevent the sufferings around us. The wellsprings of primordial compassion rise in us constantly to dissolve the limits we have set for ourselves and our view of the world.

The renowned biologist, Scott Gilbert, has taken pains to demonstrate how much of our human body, fate, and identity are reliant on genes and processes recognized to be human.

"We have about 160 major species of bacteria in our bodies, and they all form complex ecosystems. Human bodies are and contain a plurality of ecosystems. Our mouths are different ecosystems than our intestines, or our skin or our airways. The volume of the microbial organisms in our bodies is about the same as the volume of our brain, and the metabolic activity of those microbes is about equivalent to that of our liver…we are not *anatomically* individuals at all.

"(The) alleged genetic basis of individuality is scientifically wrong. The symbionts (non-genetically human micro-organisms in the human body) are another mode of (our) inheritance. Indeed, while humans have about 22,000 different genes, the bacteria in us bring approximately 8 million more genes to the scene. We get our symbionts primarily by infection from the mother as we pass through the birth canal after the amnion breaks. These bacteria are supplemented by those from the mother's skin and from the environment."

Thus our life is interwoven with, and dependent on, many more non-human than human genetic offspring. Scott concludes that we are not individuals by any biological, physiological, developmental, genetic, or evolutionary criteria. As he puts it: "Symbiosis is the strategy that supports life on earth… it is the way of life on earth."

From believing that we are single, unitary, independent beings, we view the world as for or against us. From clinging to our survival, to the survival of our world, and adhering to the specific concepts believed to support them, come all the fears of those who wage aggressive war, and the pitiful terrors of those who are war's victims. From this single source comes the predatory search for wealth, the sufferings of poverty, the longings of passion, and the ceaseless dissatisfactions of restlessness.

And with these emotional states comes the logic devoted to their perpetuation. Thus our inner lives become circumscribed by the vicious defensive logic of warfare, the economic logic of need, the lonely logic of relationships, the calculating logic of ambition. And we live a life of anxiety and confusion as we try to find our way amid the competing claims and conflicts of these logics.

Caught by anxiety about our own future, we only appreciate those beings, things, and expressions which further our version of survival. The rest of the world seems shadowy, threatening, or possibly helpful, depending on its congruence with our own conceptions.

We can regard other beings only according to whatever logic we have adopted as necessary to our happiness. Thus we come to believe that the world is populated with beings whose view of life is inimical to us, and with a far smaller group whose explicit goals and aspirations we share. We evaluate all the world around us in this way. We judge rain, sunlight, wind, and stones according to their utility in our scheme of things.

Such an outlook is not so much a departure from the spontaneous expanse of great compassion as an attempt to limit it. The sufferings we experience, and those we cause, all arise from the effort to reduce and categorize the overwhelming diversity of experience into the single framework of our own survival and posterity.

In a glimpse of the vastness and depth of the great compassion without reference point, we see mirrored the terrible and ferocious pettiness which has masqueraded as individual grandiosity and reasonableness. We see our own inescapable craven clinging. We see how we and all others are prisoners of our own individuality. We may have some choice in whether to perpetuate this condition, but we did not choose or create this delusory clinging in the first place.

In the Avatamsaka Sutra, it is said:

...all worlds
Vast and small,
One body, countless lands;
One land, countless bodies.
...
The compassionate
Comprehend their becoming and decay
Of the numberless lands
Of past, present, and future.

Of all the worlds in the ten directions,
Some are forming, some decaying:
Infinite though they be,
The truly compassionate comprehend them all.

§ § §

In any given instant, no matter what our own individual suffering, if we sit still and look around us, it is evident that we are always the recipients of an infinite array of man-made and natural phenomena. We may glimpse the limitless compassion which is itself spontaneous, unfabricated, free from concepts or views of any kind. We have the solidity of earth within and below our bodies; we have the cooling clarity of water; we have the warmth of fire and the movement of wind; we have an infinity of space articulated as sky or imagination. We have the perceptions of sight, sound, touch, taste, and smell, all as vivid as a shimmering rainbow of light. We have unending primordial awareness. And through all the realms of life and death, there is the ceaseless pulse of life force.

We have no existence apart from this array, nor are we independent from the ways of thinking, feeling, and knowing about our world, which have been developed by countless others before us. We carry out our daily lives in reliance on language evolved and wisdom discovered by others, inspiration fostered by others, laws enacted by others, information, opinions, and expressions derived from others, art created by others, technologies created by others, machines and houses made by others, energy produced by others, and food grown by others. There has never been a minute in our lives in which we have not relied on the efforts of many other people. We cannot exist independent of the lives of millions of viruses, microscopic organisms, molds, plants, insects, fish, reptiles, animals.

Nor is it possible to act in such a way that others are not influenced or affected by what we do. On a purely psychological level, even our most private thoughts and feelings inevitably influence our outer moods and our behavior. Sadness hangs in the air; private irritation turns into a more general atmosphere of tension; enthusiasm is infectious. However we are stirred up moves the air around us, touches even strangers. When we see a dog stretch in the sun, an old man stumble, a child lose her temper, or lovers touch, we too are moved, and we carry that movement into whatever comes next.

And when it comes to our standards of living which we long ago took for granted, it is now all too clear that the material bases for our daily life, from computers to toothbrushes, have a huge impact on the planet. Our food, clothes, transportation, housing, information, all are supported by a network of energy usages that cannot be sustained. The environment may already be so compromised that it will not support a similar life for our children and children's children.

Thus, regardless of whether we are kind or ruthless, selfish or generous, we live in an immeasurable ocean of phenomena that arise from our interdependence with an inconceivable range of other phenomena. We might wish to have individual autonomy and to be independent of the world we find ourselves in, but this is not in any way realistic.

When we open our hearts and rest in the free expanse of what is given in our lives, we meet the vast mind of primordial compassion which goes far beyond any individual preoccupation, belief, or fear. All our unique and individual efforts are simply part of this endless and anonymous outpouring. We sense our unconditional linkage with this world, and with all who dwell and have dwelt here. Complete openness in this way is the experience of compassion without reference point.

Even as the expanse of great compassion is without limit, calculation, or bias, the experience of it is not necessarily comforting. Though we may recognize that we are completely reliant on this world and its history, the world will not necessarily confirm us, give us what we want, or bring everything we have striven for to a successful conclusion. Even though we may find ourselves unaccountably happy in unsought moments, still we may not be able to find meaningful work, make those who love us happy, or keep our children safe. Except momentarily, we will not be saved from death, nor will we be able to save anyone else from death.

Trungpa Rinpoche grew up and was trained in remote eastern Tibet. His principal teacher was Jamgön Kongtrül of Sechen, a hard bitten, no-nonsense mountain man. Despite his harshness, Trungpa Rinpoche had complete faith that Kongtrül was teaching him not just words, but a deeper truth. Nonetheless, there was a time when Rinpoche, who was maybe nine or ten at the time, felt caught up in doubt and resentment. Sechen Kongtrül took him for a long walk in the mountains, and Trungpa Rinpoche went along begrudgingly. With every step he felt more wretched. Finally, Kongtrül stopped and they rested. Trungpa Rinpoche couldn't let go of feeling completely and stubbornly alone. They sat for quite a while until Kongtrül turned to him. "Do you love me?" he asked.

At that, as Rinpoche later said, something broke open inside him, and he sobbed uncontrollably. He understood something that had eluded him until then. On the sole occasion when he told this story, it was to point at the unsparingly personal dimension at the heart of the entirety of Buddhist teachings.

The three aspects of compassion are actually and completely inseparable. They are not exterior to us, and thus, the teachings themselves are an expression of that love.

In the face of real suffering and continual frustration, we feel a separation which we strive to understand and justify. At the same time, we also feel, however awkwardly, a wave of deep and inescapable connectedness. At the edge of awareness, we sense that every moment of our life moves within a kind of vast, luminous pulse, uncomfortably free and freeing from all limits of any kind. Inseparable from the ever-changing dance of phenomena, it is stable. Unwavering, it arises within all the displays of temporary circumstance.

In this world where pollution, continuing isolation, uncertainty, selfishness, conflict, and fear vie in our minds with the loftiest aspirations and longing, compassion is the path which represents the innate unity of relative appearance and ultimate truth. As such, compassion is not a path which is undertaken because it leads somewhere else. It does not lead to an escape or transcendence of the world, nor does it lead to some form of worldly happiness per se. It does not require the rejection of our daily experience, nor the rejection of our yearning for ultimate reality. All that we encounter, all that we experience, is this path. Compassion is not a way of living, but is living itself.

————AFTERWORD

In my early twenties I lived in New York. It was the late 1960s, a time of upheaval, fertility, surprise, unsought intensities, doubt. I did not know how to enter, to become a part of it, or what to enter or be part of. I walked the streets. One bright early summer midday, I was walking in the dappled fragrant shadows of ginkgo trees lining the street on my right and the cool marble façades of private mansions to my left. A car horn honked. A black limousine was parked just ahead. I looked, and the dark rear window slid down.

A woman, very young, her face elaborately made up, peach-colored cheeks, shining dark lips, hair in ringlets, her jade eyes with long eyelashes gazed out at me. I was stunned. I had never seen such allure. She seemed to shimmer slightly. She seemed to be from somewhere else. She stared gravely, waiting. I was paralyzed. Then the window closed back up, and the limo pulled smoothly away.

I never knew what I should have done, if I should have done anything. It was a moment whose resonance stayed and drew me on. It was a lyrical sensation shaping my longing, my uncertainty, and how I continued wandering through the city, especially at night. It was a promise of some new search, and some new and unimagined intimacy, some new and unimagined world.

Seeking does not wane. The persistent intuition that there is something just beyond the limit of the senses, on the far side of the edge of the known, is ever unassuaged. And promising, and alluring, and fearsome. It is the ever-seeking heart. No doubt this is what the sages of long ago meant when they said that mind or heart/mind is that which seeks an object. They, who took refuge in forests or desert monasteries, and we, with all our electronic gear, cars, and packaged supermarket food, are linked. We all are still searching.

Now for us, however, the path has swerved. Quarantined, our routines have been curtailed. In an environment where a virus may take us unannounced, we venture out only with great caution. We no longer touch. Our smiles are hidden beneath our masks. Our personal communications are largely online and two-dimensional. No one travels. Our driving is limited. Reliant on the media in our solitude, we are more intensely aware of the winds of manipulation.

Except for doing what we need to do each day, nothing is so demanding, so urgent. Without the press of work and time, we are anxious and unmoored. We don't know what to expect. We don't know how to think of it. We have less to distract us, and less to focus on. Things simplify themselves.

And the sky without airplanes is suddenly still. Roads without traffic are silent. An underlying silence emerges. The air, suddenly, is clearer. Bird song is louder. Mountain lions, bears, deer, and foxes are seen in the street. New green leaves are bright. Distant mountains become visible. Colors of trees, grasses, streams, and clouds are sharply brilliant. Pollution abates, and the earth flourishes. It is a cold spring. Outer stillness meets with inner. It is not entirely comfortable.

Now we see clearly how our way of life, with its toilet paper, cars, ordinary luxuries of travel and cruises, our mass-produced food and goods transported from afar, all this is dulling our lives and fouling the earth. And when we are forced to stop, how quickly, how vividly things recover.

But the price clearly is much too high. The impoverishment, the homelessness, the starvation, the sickness, and the mass suffering that arise with this is impossible to perpetuate or endure. We must return to our old ways as soon as we can. "Get back to normal," is the cry. But the old normal can no longer offer such security. It is falling apart before our eyes. And when did the past ever return?

There are no longer universally accepted opinions and unquestioned conventional truths. Mass violence has begun. With so many unemployed across the world, so many industries silenced, so many restaurants, shoe shops, small service businesses shuttered, with riots and looting in so many major cities, with nakedly brutal and self-seeking lies being broadcast from the summit of government, the world seems suddenly on the verge of imploding.

I remember the time I was descending on an escalator into the baggage area of Newark airport. I saw my father's feet (he was justly proud of his shoes) and then legs on the floor. They were sticking out from a standing crowd of policemen and EMTs. They were urgently trying to revive him, but he was dying. I wanted simply not to see it or not be part of it, or to have it not happen. I wanted to go backwards. But I was on an escalator carrying me into this new and fatherless present. And so it is now. We are being carried forward into a disturbed and disturbing unknown. We must move forward.

"Oh," we realize. "This has been going on for a long time." We hadn't noticed. Or wanted to notice. But now we must. A new world that has not yet quite shown itself is emerging.

In vain we look for clues. Outside us, we sense that reason, faith in reason, is eroding. Things feel less solid, more strange. "We are in this together," says the sign. But we feel, each of us, newly alone. We are adrift and wandering amid lies and lost certainties. We feel, even in the solitude of our own homes, foreigners.

Unmoored, untethered in such a torrent of change, it is easy to forget that this has forever been the world's condition. Now, once again, we must re-examine our life in the world. We must look further into ourselves to find how to proceed.

Three thousand years ago, the sages of ancient China sought to depict every moment in the process of change, from creation to destruction, in the Book of Changes, the I Ching. An extraordinary ambition.

The section called "The Wanderer" focuses on the recognition that one is now in an unfamiliar world and must be careful not to take laws and customs for granted, not to believe that one understands situations which are unfamiliar, and not to indulge in unwarranted swings of mood.

The wanderer is "clear minded and cautious" and "succeeds through smallness."

Thus, the commentaries say:

"Keeping still and adhering to clarity…success in small things. Perseverance brings success to the wanderer."

…

"'The wanderer dwells in shelter'
but has not yet obtained a place."

…

"The heart/mind of the wanderer is not at ease."

"(An empty) bird's nest burns.
At first, the wanderer laughs,
Then laments and weeps."

This is now our world. We are part of this and can't separate ourselves from any of it. We must look carefully within ourselves. We can't turn away. As so much is lost, so much that is ancient returns, so much that is new appears.

————NOTES

FOREWORD
P. 9 *"We have been living in a blind alley..."*
Victor Serge, tr. Sedgewick and Paizis, *Memoirs of A Revolutionary,*
New York Review of Books, 2012

P. 10 *"It was the human longing to connect..."*
Robert Karjel, tr. Nancy Pick, *The Swede,* Harper Collins, 2015
p.245

P. 11 *"Just take a little leap after that. ... That's it!"*
Chogyam Trungpa Rinpoche, *Glimpses of Realization,* Vajradhatu
Publications, 2003, p.80

A WORLD EVER AT ITS END
P. 14 *"Cold prickles my scalp..."*
Osip Mandelstam, tr. Deborah Marshall and Douglas Penick, Agni,
April, 2013

P. 17 *"Death loomed up once again..."*
Jorge Semprun, tr. Linda Coverdale, *Literature or Life,* Viking Press,
1997, pp.16

P. 18 *"I saw two villages, one on this side..."*
Erik Mueggler, *The Age of Wild Ghosts,* University of California
Press, 2001, p.175

P. 18 *"Simple and self-assured, the singer..."*
Hans Erich Nossack, tr. Joel Agee, *The End,* University of Chicago
Press, 2004, pp.51-2

P. 19 *"We need to lose the world..."*
Hélène Cixous, tr. Cornell and Sellars, *Three Steps On The Ladder
of Writing,* Columbia University Press, 1993, p.10

A VANISHED BUDDHIST KING

The following sources were invaluable in the completion of this chapter. Special thanks to these extraordinary scholars for their path-breaking work:

Vello Vaartnou, *Lubsan Samdan Tsydenov, Bidya Dandaron and The Abbot of Kumbum*

Nikolay Tsyrempilov, *Samdan Tsydenov And His Buddhist Theocratic Project in Siberia*, Chinese Buddhist Encyclopedia, p.5-9

Luboš Belka, *Mandala and History*, Masaryk University Press, 2016, p.49

FOUR DIVINE MESSENGERS: OLD AGE

This Siddhartha retelling is extensively adapted from *The Life of Buddha*, by A. Ferdinand Herold, tr. by Paul C Blum, 1922, at sacred-texts.com pp.42-44

FOUR DIVINE MESSENGERS: SICKNESS

This Siddhartha retelling is extensively adapted from *The Life of Buddha*, by A. Ferdinand Herold, tr. by Paul C Blum, 1922, at sacred-texts.com pp.44-46

P. 63-66
Wikipedia, List of Distinct Cell Types

P. 69 "Stranger within me, stranger at my side..."
Artur Lundquist, tr. A. Weissman and A. Planck, *Journeys In Dream And Imagination*, Four Walls Eight Windows, 1991, p.126.

FOUR DIVINE MESSENGERS: DEATH

This Siddhartha retelling is extensively adapted from The Life of Buddha, by A. Ferdinand Herold, tr. by Paul C Blum, 1922, at sacred-texts.com pp.46-8

P. 74
Margaret W. Morton, *Cities of the Dead: The Ancestral Cemeteries of Kyrgyzstan*, University of Washington Press, 2014

PP. 80-81
Syama Sangit 190, tr. Rachel McDermott, *Bengali Songs to Kali* from *Religions of India in Practice*, Princeton University Press 1995, p.66

FOUR DIVINE MESSENGERS: PATH

This Siddhartha retelling is extensively adapted from The Life of Buddha, by A. Ferdinand Herold, tr. by Paul C Blum, 1922, at sacred-texts.com, pp.56-9

P. 91 *"When moving through reality, like space..."*
Matthew Kapstein , *Dohas and Gray Texts: Reflections on a Song Attributed to Kanha*, www.academia.edu, p.297

P. 91 *""The goal exists in every moment of our life..."*
Chogyuam Trungpa Rinpoche, *Crazy Wisdom Seminar,* 1972: Uncredited Transcript, Talk 1, p.2-3; Talk 2, p.2

DIE GLEISE (THE TRACKS)

PP. 104-105: Adapted from Giovanni Boccaccio, tr. Musa & Bondanlella, *The Decameron*, Norton Press, 1977, pp.4-6

PATHS IN GATHERING DARKNESS

These sources were invaluable in the completion of this chapter:

Tilopa's *Mahamudra Upadesha,* from *The Life of the Mahasiddha Tilopa*, Mar-pa Chos-kyi-blo-gros, Mar-pa, tr. Fabrizio Torricelli and Sans-rgyas-bstan-dar, Library of Tibetan Works and Archives, 1995

Sangyes Nyenpa, tr. David Molk, *Tilopa's Mahamudra Upadesha: The Gangama Instructions with Commentary*, Shambhala Publications, 2014

Wikipedia, Tilopa's Six Precepts or Words of Advice

P. 122 "The elements do not have the essential nature..."
Wangchuk Dorje, tr. Tyler Dewar, *Feast for the Fortunate*, Snowlion Books, p.311

THE EMPTY BOAT
PP. 125-127
The Lotus Sutra, tr. B. Watson, Columbia University Press, 1993

P. 129 *"Perhaps it is not-being that is the true state..."*
Marcel Proust, tr. Kilmartin and Moncrieff, *Swann's Way*

P. 88 *"Birth is just like riding in a boat..."*
Moon in a Dewdrop: Writings of Zen Master Dogen, tr. Brown and Tanahashi, North Point Press, 1985, p.85

A VANISHED SAGE: BIDYA DANDARON
These sources were invaluable in the completion of this chapter:

Alexandre Andreyev, *Dreams of a Pan-Mongolian State: Sandan Tsydenov, Baron Ungern, Agvan Dorjiev, Nicholas Roerich*, 2008, found at www.budcon.com

Luboš Bêlka, *Dandaron Mandala: Unofficial Buryat Sangha during the Soviet Era*, University of Latvia, Oriental Studies 2013, vol 793, pp.132-143

Wikipedia, Bidya Dandaron

Nikolay Tsyrempilov, *The Buryat Lamas at the Interface Between Two Empires*, Lecture at Indiana University, Bloomington.

Vello Vaartnou, *Lubsan Samdan Tsydenov, Bidya Dandaron and The Abbot of Kumbum*, www.academia.edu

Alexander Piatigorsky, "The Departure of Dandaron," *Kontinent 2,* Anchor Books, 1977, p.177

Bidya Dandaron: Thoughts of a Buddhist, Moscow, 1970, provisional tr. Deborah Marshall and DJ Penick, p.3

Vladimir Montlevich, *Is There A Point In Talking About Vajrasattva?* from www.budcom.com

FOR MUSIC

PP. 147-148 *"...in an instant of awareness..."*
Avatamsaka (Flower Ornament) Sutra, 1403

P. 148 *"Night Rain at Kuang-k'ou"*
Yang Wan Li, tr. Jonathan Chaves, *Heaven My Blank, Earth My Pillow,* White Pine Press, 2004, p.123

P. 149 *"Gerald de Barri, a 12th-century Welsh churchman..."*
Richard Taruskin, Music from the Earliest Notations To The Sixteenth Century – Oxford University Press, 2010, p.147

P. 149 *"the voices remain independent..."*
Mikhail Bakhtin, *Problems of Dostoevsky's Poetics,* tr. Caryl Emerson, University of Minnesota,1984, p.21

P. 151 *"Many histories come together here..."*
5)Anna Laubenhaupt Tsing, *The Mushroom at the End of the World,* Princeton University Press, 2015, pp.157-8

P. 152 *"selves exist simultaneously..."*
Eduardo Kohn, *How Forests Think,* University of California Press, 2013, p.106 and P.19

P. 153 *"the captured ambiences — rich textures..."*
Bernie Krause, *The Great Animal Orchestra,* Little Brown and Company, 2012, e-book loc. 473

P. 153 "wandering in the pain of this cyclical illusion..."
MKV(P) p. 536 KKV(V)p.236; cit. in *Nagarjuna: The Philosophy of the Middle Way*, D.J. Kalupahana, SUNY University Press, 1983 pp. 365-6, retranslated)

THE NOBLE HEART OF EXISTENCE
P. 162 *"We have about 160 major species..."*
Scott Gilbert, "Holobiont By Birth" from *Arts of Living on Damaged Planet*, p.75

P. 164 *"...all worlds/ Vast and small..."*
Modified from *The Flower Ornament Scripture*, vol.II, tr. Thomas Cleary, Shambhala Publications, 1986, p.272

AFTERWORD
P. 172 *"Keeping still and adhering to clarity..."*
The I Ching – Book of Changes, tr. Richard Wilhem and Cary Baynes, Princeton University Press, 1950, PP. 675-678

——ACKNOWLEDGEMENTS

It is due to the kindness, thoughtfulness, generosity, hard work and, ultimately, faith of Askold Melnyczuk and Ezra Fox of Arrowsmith Press that *The Age of Waiting* now sees the light of day. Their care and detailed attention have brought it to a more evolved and much clearer form than would otherwise ever have happened. I am everlastingly grateful.

This book also could never have been written without the inspiration and support of James Shaheen and Emma Varvaloukas at *Tricycle Magazine* where more than half these pieces first appeared. Thanks also to the editors and staff at the *Shambhala Sun*, now *Lion's Roar*, for publishing two pieces, and to Catherine Parnell at *Consequence Magazine*, a journal on the culture of war.

In everything here, whether near or far, Chögyam Trungpa Rinpoche is active in the background.

Many people have patiently reviewed these pieces, first and foremost my wife, Deborah Marshall, and my good friend, Kidder Smith. Among other friends whose encouragement has been especially sustaining are Emilio Ambasz, Genny Kapular, Gianni Longo, Zentatsu Richard Baker, Ken Green, the late Martin Fritter, the late Peter Serkin, and Meg Federico.

The Age of Waiting has been produced with kind assistance from Emilio Ambasz and the Ambasz Foundation.

Thank you all so much.

DJP
Boulder, CO

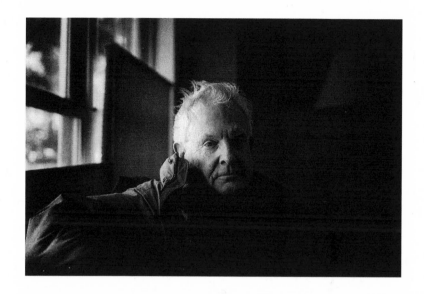

DOUGLAS J. PENICK has written opera libretti (Munich Biennale, Santa Fe Opera), texts for video (NFB/Canada: Leonard Cohen, narrator), as well as novels on the 3rd Ming Emperor (*Journey of the North Star*) and about spiritual searchers (*Dreamers and Their Shadows*). He also wrote three book-length episodes from the Gesar of Ling epic on a grant for the Witter Bynner Foundation. Wakefield Press published his and Charles Ré's translation of Pascal Quignard's *A Terrace In Rome*. Shorter works appeared in *Agni, Chicago Quarterly, Cahiers de L'Herne, New England Quarterly, Kyoto Journal, Tricycle, Utne Reader*, and many others.

ARROWSMITH is named after the late William Arrowsmith, a renowned classics scholar, literary and film critic. General editor of thirty-three volumes of *The Greek Tragedy in New Translations*, he was also a brilliant translator of Eugenio Montale, Cesare Pavese, and others. Arrowsmith, who taught for years in Boston University's University Professors Program, championed not only the classics and the finest in contemporary literature, he was also passionate about the importance of recognizing the translator's role in bringing the original work to life in a new language.

Like the arrowsmith who turns his arrows straight and true,
a wise person makes his character straight and true.

— Buddha

Books by
ARROWSMITH
PRESS

Girls by Oksana Zabuzhko
Bula Matari/Smasher of Rocks by Tom Sleigh
This Carrying Life by Maureen McLane
Cries of Animal Dying by Lawrence Ferlinghetti
Animals in Wartime by Matiop Wal
Divided Mind by George Scialabba
The Jinn by Amira El-Zein
Bergstein edited by Askold Melnyczuk
Arrow Breaking Apart by Jason Shinder
Beyond Alchemy by Daniel Berrigan
*Conscience, Consequence: Reflections on
Father Daniel Berrigan* edited by Askold Melnyczuk
Ric's Progress by Donald Hall
Return To The Sea by Etnairis Rivera
The Kingdom of His Will by Catherine Parnell
Eight Notes from the Blue Angel by Marjana Savka
Fifty-Two by Melissa Green
Music In—And On—The Air by Lloyd Schwartz
Magpiety by Melissa Green
Reality Hunger by William Pierce
Soundings: On The Poetry of Melissa Green edited by Sumita Chakraborty
The Corny Toys by Thomas Sayers Ellis
Black Ops by Martin Edmunds
Museum of Silence by Romeo Oriogun
City of Water by Mitch Manning
Passeggiate by Judith Baumel
Persephone Blues by Oksana Lutsyshyna
The Uncollected Delmore Schwartz edited by Ben Mazer
The Light Outside by George Kovach
The Blood of San Gennaro by Scott Harney edited by Megan Marshall
No Sign by Peter Balakian
Firebird by Kythe Heller
The Selected Poems of Oksana Zabuzhko edited by Askold Melnyczuk